MASTER SECRETS
of
HYPNOSIS
and
SELF-HYPNOSIS

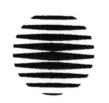

MASTER SECRETS
of
HYPNOSIS
and
SELF-HYPNOSIS

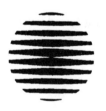

Professor Kurt Tepperwein

Instant Improvement, Inc.

Originally published in German as *Die Hohe Schule der Hypnose*,
© 1977 by Ariston Verlag, Geneva
© 1991, English version, Edi-Inter & Athena
    Copyright, London

Instant Improvement, Inc.
210 E. 86th Street, Suite 501
New York, New York 10028

Printed in the United States of America

Library of Congress Catalog Card Number: 91-73801

ISBN 0-941683-15-X

CONTENTS

VOLUME ONE
MASTER SECRETS OF
DISCOVERING HYPNOSIS

VOLUME TWO
MASTER SECRETS OF
PRACTICING HYPNOSIS ON OTHERS

VOLUME THREE
MASTER SECRETS OF
UNDETECTABLE HYPNOSIS ON OTHERS

VOLUME FOUR
MASTER SECRETS OF SELF-HYPNOSIS

This book is intended as a reference only, not a medical manual or guide to self-treatment. If you suspect you have a medical problem, we urge you to seek competent medical help. Information here is not to be used as a substitute for any treatment that may have been prescribed by your doctor.

Volume I

Master Secrets of Discovering Hypnosis

EDITOR'S NOTE

You are now in possession of the complete system, *Master Secrets of Hypnosis and Self-Hypnosis*, by Prof. Kurt Tepperwein. It is — to my knowledge — the most complete practical system that has appeared to date, and I congratulate you on your choice.

The major difference between a system and a book is — aside from the quality and unusualness of the information revealed — the way it is absorbed, and its practical aspect.

Prof. Kurt Tepperwein, an eminent practitioner of hypnosis, will lead you step by step through the Universe of the Mind. This fascinating exploration should not be taken lightly. Take all the time necessary to thoroughly absorb the new ideas and techniques which will be presented.

Don't hesitate to provide yourself with a pencil and eraser and to take notes from each page. Copy them onto cards. Memorize them. The texts of the hypnotic suggestions you should learn are printed in *large italics*. If it will help you, you may also copy these into a notebook, or dictate them into a tape recorder.

This system is presented in as simple and direct a manner as possible. Prof. Tepperwein will help you master the theory of hypnosis at the same time as its practice. His method is simple and will require little effort — only perseverance.

To derive all the benefits of the system, don't think of it as a novel, and try to resist the inclination to "devour" it as quickly as possible.

Just as travelling on foot allows you to enjoy the countryside more than by automobile, examine every detail. Then make sure that you have thoroughly understood it before going on to the next step.

If you wish, you may begin by reading this first volume all at once, on condition that this first reading be an orientation that prepares you for the real work of assimilation.

In this case, work through each volume one after the other, and do not go on to volume 2 before thoroughly mastering volume 1.

Or, if you wish, start with volume 4, on self-hypnosis. Prove the amazing powers on yourself first, before you try them on anyone else.

Throughout, you will learn by putting into practice. There is no need for you to be satisfied with only intellectual knowledge. You will retain it far better by putting it at once into practical use, and your experiences will cause you to raise questions that will lead you back to the system.

With *Master Secrets of Hypnosis and Self-Hypnosis*, you will be taken in hand by a Master who will pass on to you everything that years of practice and experience have taught him.

Even if certain passages seem too simple to be true, even if certain ideas are contrary to your personal convictions, put your trust in him. Prof. Tepperwein does not ask you to believe in his word. He asks you to prove everything for yourself.

But do remember that Hypnosis is a field in which positive thinking is all important! Therefore, your doubts will be magnified: cast them aside. Your fears will retard your progress: refuse to give heed to them.

Do not hesitate to proceed from the easiest of these hypnotic accomplishments to the most complex. Set a series of ever-growing objectives for yourself. Gain courage as you progress. And remember, if you receive a setback, reread this sentence:

To become a true master of the techniques of hypnosis, you must practice, practice and practice yet again.

But I can feel your impatience to get going on the adventure. I must admit to being a little envious of the elation you will experience in the weeks and months to come. What indeed can be more fascinating than hypnosis?

It will lead you to the discovery of the most secret workings of the human organism.

It will guide you towards true knowledge of yourself.

It will allow you to bring to light the strength, the self-confidence and the mastery which are today only potentially in you — and which will give you the ability to radically transform your life.

Happy travelling, and all my wishes for Success!

Christian H. Godefroy

Editor

PREFACE

By Prof. Helmut Jansen

This system, *Master Secrets of Hypnosis and Self-Hypnosis*, has been written following *Geistheilung Durch Sich Selbst (Psychokybernetik, Hypnomeditation)*, by Prof. Tepperwein. This method is a practical teaching manual. The author, director of the International Institute for Research and Development of Hypnosis, has made his work accessible to both amateurs and practitioners. All the secrets of hypnotic technique are discussed. After studying the method, you will be able to practice hypnosis on others and on yourself. You will be able to acquire experience by putting them into practice.

Thanks to self-hypnosis, you will develop your positive qualities and correct your faults. The hypnosis of others is an effective means of coming to the aid of your fellow man. But if, through hypnosis, you wish to dominate the latter, you have not grasped the essence of it.

The first step towards wisdom is to want to have an accurate assessment of one's personal worth. Put yourself honestly to the test. Consider the result of this self-analysis as a step along the road to perfection, for your "I" is already potentially perfect.

Rio de Janeiro, March 1977

> Prof. Dr. Med. Helmut Jansen
> Dean of the Faculty of Medicine,
> Santa Ursula University,
> Rio de Janeiro, Brazil.

HOW TO SUCCEED WITH EVERY HYPNOSIS AND SELF-HYPNOSIS

I would like to set out for you a brief summary of the various phases and conditions required to succeed with hypnosis.

THE CONDITIONS

The essential condition is that you believe in yourself.

He who does not believe in himself cannot expect to gain the confidence of someone else. An atmosphere of confidence on the patient's part, and sympathy on your part, is of prime necessity.

Once you have established the right atmosphere for your office – once you have made it comfortable, welcoming, and shielded from the distractions of the outside world – you can put the following questions to the patient.

"Have you ever been hypnotized? By what method?"

If the answer is yes, you then know what method has been effective with this patient, or ineffective with him. If it has, you have an automatic head start. If it has not, avoid that method at all costs.

If he has not been hypnotized, proceed as follows:

First of all, all misbeliefs, all false hopes that he brings with him, must be eliminated.

For example, many people confuse hypnosis with trance. They imagine that the hypnotic state is total unconsciousness. Hypnotism may then disappoint them, and they will not be able to get what they want from a light stage of hypnosis.

So tell the patient that hypnosis is a natural state. Every individual is regularly in this state: when we fall asleep, on awakening, etc. . . . Under hypnosis, nothing unusual takes place.

Next, find out the desires which led the patient to consult you. Here are some standard questions:

"What is your main desire?"

"What is your basic problem?"

The replies to these questions are in general very instructive.

HOW DO YOU FORMULATE THE HEALING SUGGESTIONS?

Once you have obtained the necessary information, begin to formulate your suggestions.

First, give a logical order to the desires . . then transform them into effective and positive suggestions.

Try not to say, "Now, you have no more headaches".

Suggest instead, "Your head is clear, free of all pain".

Once your suggestions are formulated, create a positive tension in his mind due to his expectation of being healed. Make him *want* to give control to you, because he can begin to see that you are the source of the fulfillment of his dreams.

Reassure the patient as to your intentions, your desire to help him. Explain that hypnosis will resolve all his problems. The patient must want the hypnotic state.

Such preparation excludes all resistance and will encourage a beneficial influence.

METHODS USED TO HELP THE PATIENT

The patient, with his eyes closed, rests for ten to thirty minutes in a quiet, dimly-lit room. Soft music will reinforce this feeling of peace. The room's colors will preferably be green or blue.

The only means employed by a good hypnotist will be his voice, and the influence exerted by his personality.

Here is a simple method, infallible and very effective.

Hang a quarter from the ceiling, slightly above the patient's eyes. He will look at it. His eyes will eventually close.

HOW IS HYPNOSIS INDUCED?

Build your positive suggestions on the information he has given you.

Choose a hypnotic technique that weaves this information into a logical stream of suggestions that gently – step by step – achieve the desires of the patient.

Your tone of voice will be calm, its rhythm measured. Create vivid, detailed mental images that you can then implant in his subconscious.

Do not be in a hurry. Give the images as much detail as they demand. Repeat them again and again, as you see them taking effect in his answers to your questions or his actions. As he progresses, intensify the hypnosis by suggesting that he sink into one deeper level after another.

Do not forget that your voice contains two separate elements, tone and content. Both must be in harmony with each other.

Here is an obvious example. If you suggest: "You are quite calm and relaxed", in a nagging, peremptory tone, you will achieve an opposite effect.

Adapt your suggestions to the intellectual level of the patient as well. Seek to identify wholly with him during the hypnosis. This requires complete concentration. But without this total assimilation, you cannot transfer the influence exerted by your personality to the patient.

THE STEPS BY WHICH YOU MANAGE A HYPNOSIS

First stage: physical relaxation.

You will obtain it from these phrases:

"You are lying comfortably . . . Your eyes are closed . . . Your arms and legs are flexible . . . Relaxed . . . You are breathing slowly, evenly . . . With each breath, you sink deeper and deeper and deeper . . . etc. . . . "

Second stage: psychic relaxation.

"You no longer want anything . . . Be passive . . . Let yourself go . . . Let it be . . . Let it hap-

*pen . . . Nothing distracts
you . . . Your head is clear . . .
etc . . . "*

Third stage: peace and well-being.

*"You rejoice in this sense of well-
being that envelops you from head
to foot . . . Feel this wonderful
relaxation which spreads more and
more throughout your body . . .
etc . . . "*

Fourth stage: creating an opening to the subconscious.

*" . . . In this wonderful state of
peace, you have an opening to the
subconscious . . . A wider and
wider opening . . . Your subconscious is registering all my
words . . . They are deeply engraved there . . . You will
obey . . . etc . . . "*

Fifth stage: individual suggestions.

In this stage, give suggestions which have been

formulated according to the information obtained. Recorded and reordered by your subconscious, they will contain all the desires of the patient.

Sixth stage: suggestions of well-being and peace.

Repeat those of the third stage.

Seventh stage: encourage a second hypnosis.

". . . If I put you under hypnosis again, you will sink more rapidly than the previous time . . . The more hypnoses you undergo, the deeper they will be."

Eighth stage: free him from all the physical suggestions of not being able to move, etc.

Release him from all suggestions through which you caused him to sink into hypnosis. But remember, you must leave him with the suggestion that motivated the treatment.

" . . . Your arms and legs are once more flexible and capable of movement . . . Feel it. You are free, light . . . On three, you will open your eyes . . . You will feel fresh

and alert . . . One. . . Two . . .
Three . . . etc . . . "

Ninth stage: the concluding suggestion, that of well-being.

" . . . Now, you are completely awake, full of strength and energy . . . Feel it. You are fresh and alert . . . etc . . . "

HOW DO YOU CONTROL DIFFICULTIES?

1. Even the most skeptical patients can be hypnotized, if you proceed stage by stage. Refer to the appropriate chapter.

Do not be discouraged if an attempt does not immediately succeed. Questioning will allow you to discover the effective suggestions. Repeat and strength these. Avoid any negative suggestions.

If you have access to a G.S.R., you will be able to form a precise idea of the effect obtained by following the needle on the dial. You will adjust your behavior accordingly. This will give a unique character to the hypnosis.

2. Do not become panic-stricken if a patient does not immediately awaken. Deepen the hypnosis. Raise his arm and give him the following suggestion:

"As soon as I lower your arm, you will awaken . . . If I push your arm against the side of your body, you will be completely awake. You will feel in great form".

It will rarely be necessary to repeat this suggestion.

HOW DO YOU DEEPEN THE HYPNOSIS?

The most effective method remains the repetition of the suggestion.

If this procedure is insufficient, use split hypnosis.

Also give this suggestion:

"You are sinking into a deeper and deeper sleep . . . Each new sleep . . . Each new hypnosis will be deeper and deeper".

3. It would be wise to cover the person to be hypnotized. He will feel at ease, reassured. The blanket reminds him of bed and encourages sleep.

4. The effect of transference under hypnosis will be strengthened if you are yourself in a light version of this state.

5. If you are dealing with a very nervous person, produce a calming effect by massaging the reflexive zones of the bottom of his feet.

THE SUGGESTION

The suggestion is the formation, by you, of a mental image in your subconscious, which you then convey by speech to your patient. When it is formulated positively, and spoken in a pleasant tone, the patient will then transform it into a mental image in his unconscious.

Separate your suggestions into three phases:

1. "Soon, something will happen."

2. "You are feeling it happen."

3. "Now it has happened."

Here is a practical example:

1. "Your stomach is getting warm."

2. "Feel how it is getting warm."

3. "Now it is warm."

In the event of pain, suggest a sensation of warmth surging into the place concerned. Intensify and repeat the suggestion again and again. This will dissipate the suffering.

PAUSES

This is a very good procedure for deepening the suggestions given. End one phase of the hypnosis, then observe a minute of silence before inducing another. During this pause, the patient concentrates exclusively on the suggestions recorded in his subconscious. They will take greater root there.

Next, before inducing any new hypnosis, you will observe three minutes of silence.

ENDING THIS TREATMENT'S SUGGESTIONS

If you wish to dissolve a hypnotic state, first raise all the physical suggestions. Do not dissolve those which have motivated the treatment. Then suggest:

"Everything has become as it was before the hypnosis!"

START A CONVERSATION

Now question the patient on his impressions experienced under hypnosis. The information obtained will allow you to avoid, in the future, the unpleasant suggestions, and retain those which are beneficial.

Put to yourself the following questions:

"Is the patient really awake?" "Is he feeling quite well?" "Is he ready to undergo a new hypnosis?"

Check these facts.

To summarize, if you create the positive attitude in the patient described above, he will wait for the next hypnosis with pleasure.

If you follow all my advice, you are assured of success.

A SHORT HISTORY OF HYPNOSIS

ANCIENT PRACTICES OF HYPNOTISM

Historically, hypnosis began with the birth of man. Four thousand years before Christ, the Sumerians were already practicing it. This civilization, the oldest one known on earth, applied it according to certain methods still in use at the present time. Proof: the well-preserved cuneiform characters in the countries bordering the Euphrates and the Tigris.

SUMER

From time immemorial, the celebrated school for the Priests of Erech has had in its possession a manuscript, part of which has been maintained in good condition. It contains incontestable proof of cures achieved through hypnotic suggestion. One can already distinguish three gradations: light hypnosis . . . medium hypnosis . . . deep hypnosis.

INDIA

Similar gradations are represented in the book of the Law of Manu: ancient Sanskrit science of the Indian people. They are: "the sleep-waking state", "the dream-sleep", "the ecstasy-sleep".

Self-hypnosis was already used in certain yoga techniques developed in this period.

EGYPT

Ancient Egypt used hypnosis as a therapeutic measure. Its methods of application are exhibited on the Ebers Papyrus, which is three thousand years old. The procedures used are equivalent to ours. The Egyptian priests, doctors of the people, made use of their suggestive powers. Their patients stared at metal disks. The fatigue thus caused released the hypnotic sleep. The method of fixation was born.

An old Egyptian document speaks about the laying on of hands:

"Lay your hands on him ... Calm the pain in his arms and say, 'The pain will disappear ...'"

Popular sentiment attributed the cures to the gods. Those who were ill made supplications in certain temples such as that of Serapis in Canopus, and that of Isis.

GREECE

Greeks desirous of a hypnotic cure would sleep in the temples. Those who were ill would undergo a diet and special preparations: scented baths and ritual washing. Then a priest told them of previous cures. The purpose of these remarks was to stimulate "expectation", to create an atmosphere favorable to the realization of the event to come.

While they slept, the priests repeated to them the curative suggestions. These led the ill to practice autosuggestion, self-healing.

The meaning of dreams played a major part in treatment. For the Egyptian a dream meant the advice of the gods. As they concerned the mental images of suggestions made by the priests, the latter easily explained them to those who were ill. They commanded them to obey the counsel of the gods.

Insomniacs had Mediums at their disposal. These, when in hypnotic trance, entered into contact with the gods. In the celebrated temple of Delphis, consecrated to

Apollo, a priestess sat on a golden tripod, placed before a crevice in a rock. Vapors issuing from this crack were helpful for her trances. She imparted on demand the counsels of the gods. In other temples, this state was brought about by the burning of certain herbs.

For thousands of years, these priest-doctors, Sumerian and Greek, Hindu seers and yogis, made use of hypnosis.

ROME

Doctors served as intermediaries between the gods and the sick. Certain philosophers adopted the power of suggestion. The Roman poet, Porphyrus (second century A.D.), reports a conflict between two philosophers: Plotinus and Olympius.

Their pupils were arguing about the knowledge of their respective masters. Tired of the argument, Plotinus challenged Olympius to prove his gifts in "the magical art". The duel took place in the presence of the pupils of the two rivals.

Plotinus drew near Olympius, observed him for some minutes:

"Behold, his body shrivels like a purse!"

A terrible agony coursed through the body of Olympius. From that time onward, he recognized in Plotinus a mental strength superior to his own.

HYPNOSIS AND CHRISTIANITY

The application of hypnosis was replaced by religious practices in the middle of the sixth century. Christian monks had replaced the priest-doctors. New methods used were prayer, holy water, martyrs' relics, and the laying on of hands. Popes and kings referred to the New Testament to achieve "miraculous cures". It is said: "You will lay on your hands in my name, and the sick will be made whole".

In the eleventh century, monks of the Hesichastic order, cloistered on Mount Athos, inaugurated the principle of self-hypnosis. They set it in motion by gazing at their navels. Every adept of their system is called an omphalopsychic, or a contemplator of the navel.

PARACELSUS

Theophrastus Bombast of Hohenheim, known as Paracelsus (1433- 1541), taught:

"The deciding factor in a cure is the inner doctor".

He related:

"At Karnten, monks cure the sick who contemplate shining crystal balls. The patients fall into a deep sleep. Then the monks give them healing suggestions. Most of the patients come away cured".

THE INQUISITION

Under the Inquisition, this way of obtaining cures fell into oblivion. Anyone who practiced this art was declared guilty of dealing with Satan. He ran the risk of being burned alive.

FROM MAGNETISM TO SCIENTIFIC HYPNOSIS

ATHANASIUS KIRCHER (1606-1680)

In his book — *Experimentum Mirabile* — which appeared in Rome in 1646, this Jesuit father relates the "enchantment" of a cock. This first scientific treatise on the phenomenon of animal hypnosis can be considered as the forerunner of *Magnetismus Animalis* by Mesmer.

MAXIMILIAN HELL

This Jesuit father, a famous astronomer, achieved "magnetic cures". He placed "magnets", images of the diseased organ, on the painful part of the body. He obtained surprising results of 60% to 80% cures and a general improvement in condition.

FRANZ ANTON MESMER (1734-1815)

This is the father of modern hypnosis. His doctrine: The accomplishment of phenomena does not require astral magnetism, mineral magnetism, nor that of iron. The individual "Fluidum" is sufficient to magnetize the sick person. This "fluid" was transmitted by "passes" — by hand movements made from top to bottom along the body. In 1775, Mesmer sent a circular to all the well-known academics of the age. His doctrine was explained therein.

His successes and the cure of a pianist, blind from the age of four, earned him powerful enemies. He left Vienna for Paris. Among his most enthusiastic followers, let us mention Marie-Antoinette and other members of the court.

Here is his procedure. The sick, around a tub filled with magnetized water, each hold a bar of iron in their hands. The fluid causes "crises". These are transmitted by a collective contagion.

In 1784, the Academy of Sciences created, by order of King Louis XVI, a commission charged with examining the doctrine of Mesmer. This commission was made up of doctors such as Guillotin, Jolie and Sallin-D'Arcet, plus delegates from the Academy of Sciences such as Bailly, de

Bory and Lavoisier. The theory of animal fluid was dis-
credited, ridiculed. The Mesmerian cures were attributed
to the imagination. This coalition took on an international
scope. Doctors of the King of Bavaria, of the King of Den-
mark and of the Tsar of Russia were also won over.

Thus, Mesmer became the pioneer in the struggle led
by modern hypnotherapy.

ABBE FARIA (1755-1815)

This Portuguese, arriving in Paris from Goa in 1813,
laid down the theory of suggestion and refuted the Mesmerian fluid.

According to him, suggestion was enough to induce
hypnotic sleep. His book — *De la Cause du Sommeil
Lucide en Etude sur la Nature de l'Homme* — appeared in
1819. Faria called the hypnotist, "concentrator" — the one
hypnotized, "concentrated" — the hypnotic sleep, "concentration" or lucid sleep.

Here is his procedure. Place yourself very close to the
invalid. Look intently at him for a moment. . . then command, "Sleep!" 50% of patients fall into a hypnotic state.
This method precedes "Shock hypnosis" by Charcot.

JAMES BRAID (1795-1860)

This English ophthalmologist was present at experiments conducted by the magnetist La Fontaine in Manchester. Skeptical, he studied the phenomena with the sole
purpose of denouncing the deception. His patients were

his wife, his friend Walker and his servant. They gazed at a shining button set level with the bridge of the nose. Surprise! All three fell into a deep hypnotic sleep. Braid gave it the name "hypnosis" from the Greek name, hypnos, the demon of sleep.

In most cases, hypnosis occurred at the end of several minutes. No verbal suggestion was necessary. In 1842-43, his most important work appeared: *Neurohypnology or the Rationale of Nervous Sleep Considered in Relation with Animal Magnetism.* His colleagues ridiculed his doctrine.

A. A. LIÉBEAULT

This Parisian doctor examined the theories of Braid. In 1886, he published his book, *Le Sommeil Artificiel et des États Semblables.* This work did not get the attention it deserved.

HYPPOLYTE BERNHEIM (1843-1917)

Professor at the University of Nancy, he took an interest in the theories of Liébeault. He published his book, *Traité sur la Suggestion et Son Application,* in 1886. He instituted clinical hypnotherapy in Nancy.

THE SCHOOL OF NANCY

Working in collaboration with Liébeault, he created the School of Nancy. The scientific application of hypnosis was on its way.

SIGMUND FREUD

This pupil of the School of Nancy is the founder of psychoanalysis. He carried out research on hypnosis and attempted to prove its worth. His work was revived by Emile Coué and Ch. Baudouin.

EMILE COUÉ (1857-1926)

He developed the doctrine of autosuggestion: "All hypnosis is self-hypnosis". The hypnotist creates in the patient's subconscious an image of the desired effect. This is brought about by the subject himself. His maxim: "It is not the will that obliges us to act, but our imagination".

Coué deduced that each individual is a powerful hypnotist. He would say to his patients:

"Learn to cure yourself. You can do it. I have never cured anyone. This power is within you. Call on your mind for help. Make it the servant of your mental and physical well-being. It will be present; it will heal you. You will be happy".

Next, Coué directed them to repeat it twenty times morning and evening:

"Every day, in every way, I get better and better".

JEAN-MARTIN CHARCOT (1825-1893)

He was chief physician at La Salpétrière in Paris, professor of anatomy, a neurologist with a world-wide reputation. His work on nervous illnesses revolutionized the knowledge of an era.

THE PARIS SCHOOL

It was given that name by Charcot in opposition to the School of Nancy. His opinion was that "All hypnosis is an hysterical reaction". This erroneous idea was affected by the conditioning of his patients, all mentally ill. He inaugurated the "shock" technique. The means were explosion, sudden exposure to light, a gong brutally struck without any warning. The invalids, startled, fell in groups under hypnosis. His leitmotif was "Faith, alone, heals".

I.P. PAVLOV (1849-1936)

This Russian searcher discovered another aspect of hypnosis. The famous "Pavlovian dog" experiment brought about an enlightenment of psychosomatic connections. Thanks to him, hypnosis lost its mystery. According to him, hypnosis and suggestion are phenomena inherent in life.

Here is the order in which the experiment is carried out:

- ☐ Give a substantial helping of meat to a dog. Reaction obtained is a significant salivary secretion.

- ☐ Simultaneously ring a bell.

- ☐ Repeat the procedure several times.

Here is the final result that is obtained: the ringing alone will be enough to induce the secretion of saliva. Note the absence of meat. After several experiments of this type, Pavlov concluded:

"Every excitation that is recurring, long-lasting or systematic and that reaches a certain point in the neocortex, by certain nervous channels, induces a mandatory drowsiness. Sleep follows, and by extension, hypnosis".

Pavlov makes the distinction between:

- ☐ the non-conditioned reflexes which are innate.

- ☐ the conditioned reflexes acquired in the course of our lives.

His theory on conditioned reflexes allowed conclusive research to be made on the human subconscious and on the automatic functions of the higher nervous activities.

J.H. SCHULTZ

He deserves to be mentioned. His system is "Autogenous Training" from the Greek word, "autogen", generated by itself. Here is its principle: concentration and influence on oneself. The desired result is total relaxation.

Concentration in absolute stillness and self-education intensifies the depth of this relaxation. This training will allow you to mentally influence ills of a functional and organic nature, the results of inhibitions and psychic distress.

Here are the six basic exercises of Professor Schultz:

Exercise 1 — Warming up, to relax the muscles.

Exercise 2 — The sensation of warmth, to stimulate the circulation of blood.

Exercise 3 — To control the beating of the heart.

Exercise 4 — To quiet the breathing rate.

Exercise 5 — Exercising the abdominals to regulate the functions of the abdominal organs.

Exercise 6 — To produce the sensation of "cooling" of the forehead.

Positions required for execution of Autogenous Training:

1. The prone position.

2. The position called "the armchair".

3. The position called "coachman".

At the second degree of this Training, one achieves the vision of a mental image, a symbolic form of the state experienced by the subconscious.

L.M. LECRON

This American practitioner taught the techniques of hypnotherapy to thousands of physicians and psychologists. His works — *Self-Hypnosis and Heterohypnosis,* and *Self-Hypnosis* — are a collection of simple, effective procedures, accessible to the general public.

His methods eliminated the unfavorable preconceptions expressed against hypnosis.

WHAT IS HYPNOSIS?

THE BEGINNING OF YOUR PATH TO MASTERY.

AN EXAMPLE

In Tanganyika, a doctor was called to the bedside of a sick black man; the diagnosis was acute peritonitis. An operation was urgently necessary. The sick man, terror-stricken, fled to the healer of his tribe.

The healer proceeded with the customary rituals of incantations and herbs kneaded together, then applied to the painful part. The black man watched the procedure, stupefied. He did not interfere.

The healer commanded: "Feel! Your pains are gone".

Surprise! The patient returned a cured man! The medicine man had quite simply treated by suggestion under hypnosis.

THE HYPNOSIS OF OTHERS
AND SELF-HYPNOSIS

How does one define the exact nature of suggestion and hypnosis? No theory until now provides a precise statement about this.

First of all, it would be a state of semi-unconsciousness placed somewhere between sleep and the waking state.

Here are the central verified facts. Under hypnosis, physiological functions diminish, and psychic activity increases.

Here is the definition provided by the British Medical Association:

"Hypnosis is a transitory state of altered attention in the subject, a state that can be brought about by another person and in which varied phenomena can appear spontaneously or in response to oral or other stimuli.

"These phenomena include a change in consciousness and memory, an increased susceptibility to suggestion and the appearance in the subject of responses and ideas which are unfamiliar to him in his habitual frame of mind.

"Besides, phenomena such as anesthesia, paralysis, muscular rigidity and vasomotor alterations can be, in the hypnotic state, produced or suppressed". (Quotation from *L'Hypnose*, Dr. Chertok, Payot, 1969).

What is the hypnosis of others? It is the act of dictating an idea which is freely accepted by the patient.

Free consent of the subject is indispensable. This is imperative.

I conclude from this that all hypnosis is self-hypnosis, indeed even auto-suggestion. This is why it is important to repeat your idea over and over again, several times. This will generate a conditioned reflex, and will therefore become identified with the patient's personality.

LAW OF THE CONDITIONED REFLEX

Pavlov wrote:

"All unvarying and unceasing excitation which attains a point of the neo-cortex by very well-defined nerve paths, induces a mandatory sleep".

Here are the conditions necessary to obtain the best result: a quiet room, and soft lighting. The patient must not be distracted by his environment. Now, induce a hypnotic excitation, as you are shown below. Once the hypnosis is set in motion, you may then proceed to "lightning hypnosis".

LIGHTNING HYPNOSIS

This is, again, a self-hypnosis. You merely suggest the idea. This is then incorporated and applied by the patient, who produces the desired effect. Conviction and trust determine the effect. You must therefore create an atmosphere of sympathy and understanding, by means of the dialogue shown below.

EFFECTS

Reactions under hypnosis apply to every part of the person's body. Example: you can slow down or accelerate the breathing motion and the beating of the pulse. Or cause secretion of the gastric juices, sweating, coughing, vomiting, yawning, sneezing, excitement of the sexual functions, menstruation, movements of the pupil of the eye, urination and voiding of the bowels.

Illusions of the senses, either negative or positive, can equally occur under hypnosis.

AN EXAMPLE OF CONTROLLING WHAT A PATIENT WILL SEE

If you give the patient a negative suggestion, he will transform it into a false sensation. For example, he can no longer see certain objects that you say are not there.

Here is an example. Suggest to a person under hypnosis:

"You are in an empty room. Cross it!"

That person will not see the table set in the middle and will knock against it.

One day, I carried out the following experiment. I had suggested to a patient in a hypnotic state:

"You are alone in this room".

But a friend and I remained there, motionless. For a moment. Then, we started throwing soft cushions at her, to her great irritation! Her fright was such that we were obliged to stop the experiment dead.

Once she recovered from her shock, the patient recounted her impressions to us: flying cushions coming out of nowhere, what a scare!

Note her absolute conviction, under hypnosis, of having been alone in that room.

Dr. Krafft-Ebing recalls a similar experiment. He had given the suggestion:

"Dr. H. has gone away on a trip for a few days. You are quite alone!"

But Dr. H. crossed the room, a lighted cigarette in his mouth. What a shock to the patient! Terror-stricken, his eyes followed this luminous spot which seemed to move on its own. The hypnotized subject attributed this phenomenon to some magic "trick."

Another example:

You can induce temporary total blindness by simple suggestion.

Repeat the following:

"Slowly, everything is growing darker around you ... More and more ... Everything is disappearing into an impenetrable cloud ... Now, you can barely make out nearby objects ... Nothing more ... You are in total darkness".

That person will behave like a blind man. But, in such an experiment, it is necessary to expose possible pretending. To do that, place an object in the patient's path. If he is really under hypnosis, he will bump against it.

VITAL NOTE: It is important to say to the hypnotized subject:

"You will be blind for only a moment".

It is necessary to explicitly limit this blindness so as to get rid of any distress or fear that would cause the failure of the experiment.

AN EXAMPLE OF MAKING PATIENTS FOLLOW YOUR UNSPOKEN THOUGHTS

You can also do this by controlling what he will see. Here is a classic experiment using a deck of cards. Put the subject under hypnosis. Suggest:

"A black spot appears on the reverse of the card I want. Take it out of the deck".

The person will, in actual fact, remove the card you were thinking about from the deck. However, no distinctive mark was on the reverse of that card.

HYPNOSIS IS A STATE OF LIMITED CONSCIOUSNESS, WHERE THE CONSCIOUS MIND IS DOMINATED BY THE FAR GEATER POWER OF THE UNCONSCIOUS

Of course, hypnosis is very much like sleep. But do not confuse normal sleep with hypnotic sleep. During hypnotic sleep, consciousness — the too-rational part of the mind that tells us that we cannot do the "impossible" — is limited. But with hypnotic access to the unconscious, many previous "impossibilities" suddenly become possible.

According to Pavlov, in hypnosis only certain cerebral (conscious) functions would be limited, or indeed extinguished. Here is the explanation. A reduced circulation rate is equivalent to diminished cerebral activity. The functions of the higher centers of the brain, fed by capillary blood vessels, in hypnosis will be considerably lessened. The subconscious personality will come into play.

There is, in reality, a relation between sleep and the minimum of conscious perception. In a perfect resemblance, hypnosis would be no more than simple sleep.

Inhibitions are dominant in the sleeping state. Excitations take over when one is awake.

My conclusion: normal sleep is different than hypnosis.

DIFFERENCES BETWEEN HYPNOSIS AND SLEEP

THE STRUCTURE OF HYPNOSIS

1. Increased attention is attached to a suggestion received.

2. There is an awareness of every word and every noise.

3. There is lessening of the patient's critical mind.

4. There is a restricted or limited field of consciousness, although the conscious mind remains awake.

5. There is the presence of a temporary and limited sense of direction.

6. Except for a command to the contrary, the memory of the patient continues to function.

7. The hypnotized person is receptive to the spoken word.

THE STRUCTURE OF SLEEP

1. Attention is non-existent.

2. Receptivity to excitation is practically nil.

3. The critical mind is totally absent.

4. Consciousness is blocked.

5. The sense of direction is extinguished.

6. Memory is blocked.

7. The patient is no longer receptive to the spoken word.

RAPPORT

Under hypnosis, the patient's consciousness moves towards the hypnotist. A contact is created called, "rapport". The subconscious, detached from all external excitation, will faithfully record the commands of the hypnotist. You will also observe that during this rapport, the critical faculty, although clearly diminished, survives. As a result, suggestions in conflict with fundamental inclinations of the personality will immediately cancel the hypnosis.

Example:

Suggest to the patient that he disrobe or kill someone. The latter, neither exhibitionist nor assassin, will instantly awaken.

FACTORS LIKELY TO INDUCE HYPNOSIS

Remember the following:

1. Hypnosis has nothing in common with magic or supranormal phenomena.

2. Hypnosis is not artificial sleep.

3. Hypnosis is much more than mere suggestion. Suggestion is simply received and transformed more easily under hypnosis.

4. Under hypnosis, you can influence psychological illnesses, or serious organic disturbances in a positive fashion.

5. Hypnosuggestive influences are functions of the psychic activity or passivity of the person hypnotized.

6. One may suggest to the subject under hypnosis sensory illusions in either the positive or negative sense.

7. Hypnosis is not the same as sleep. But both are inherent in human and animal life.

8. Any person able to sleep is susceptible to hypnosis. The symptoms which take place during normal sleep differ from the effects produced under hypnosis.

9. Hypnosis is not, of course, a remedy for all ills. But the experienced hypnotist will find in it an effective way to help his fellow man in the best way possible.

WHAT IS SUGGESTION?

DEFINITION

Suggestion is the means of creating, in one's subconscious or in that of someone else, an image of a given idea or action. It is thus the infallible procedure for influencing other's feelings, other's judgement and other's will. If the image or idea is clear and precise, it will be easily registered. The results will be even longer-lasting.

HETEROSUGGESTION AND AUTOSUGGESTION

By heterosuggestion, we receive an idea given by another person. By autosuggestion the image is created by ourselves. But all heterosuggestion is ultimately an autosuggestion. To explain: the idea produced by the hypnotist is first engraved in the patient's subconscious . . . then is identified with . . . then is transformed into autosuggestion.

ITS REALIZATION IN THE SUBCONSCIOUS

A suggestion is never put into action by our conscious mind. It is first transformed by autosuggestion — in the subconscious mind — into a mental image of the action suggested.

The conclusion must be that all the phenomena of hypnosis are the result of suggestions or auto-suggestions.

Look at this experiment. A scholar suggests to several people:

"You are each drinking a quart of liquid".

Each person will therefore urinate a quart more than usual. However, they have all really drunk only a very little water.

How is the suggestion carried out? By inner subconscious thought. This is what generates the mental image which brings about the realization of the desired action.

It is central for you to realize that without the patient's conviction, this chain from suggestion to action is impossible. Under hypnosis, all suggestions — whether they come from you or from the patient — are accepted or refused according to the extent of our belief.

Here are other similiar factors to be taken into account:

The favorable disposition of your subject to be hypnotized.

Your power of persuasion, developed as shown below.

Your ability to change what you want into an idea that will be freely accepted by the subject. . . or into a mental image of the action you "will" in the patient's subconscious. This too will be shown to you.

WHO CAN MAKE A SUGGESTION?

Certain people master it right away. The required criteria are: great self-confidence, an outstanding personality.

Dr. Charles Baudouin remarks, "Suggestion is the unconscious realization of an idea put forward".

The psychologist Fritz Lambert states, "All suggestion is a mental influence. Believe it". We submit to it.

CONSCIOUS AND UNCONSCIOUS SUGGESTIONS

In life, we submit to certain influences from our environment, and, of course, our inner feelings influence ourselves. Thus our fate is continually determined by conscious and unconscious suggestions. Autosuggestion occupies a major place, for we take each of these ideas and incorporate it to forge our personality.

Therefore I recommend that you never forge negative ideas.

Positive and very powerful thoughts are the keys to your success.

Learn to live only with them, and eliminate all inauspicious thoughts.

THE CENTRAL RULE OF MENTAL POWER: He who knows and uses the laws of suggestion protects himself from all worries — and achieves all that he desires.

NOTE: As you have seen, for purposes of brevity, I have used the pronoun, "he", to represent both male and female. There is no sexual bias intended. Otherwise, these books would be quite awkward to read.

MAKE SUGGESTIONS THAT YOUR PATIENT CAN SEE AND THEN REALIZE

Before formulating a suggestion, try to find out if your patient is capable of reproducing a mental image of your idea. Only that of which we can form a precise image tends to be realized.

Example: Here's how to form an image of your breathing. While you inhale, imagine that you are storing up new strength. Feel the strength pouring into your body with every breath. Then feel it settling in and spreading throughout every cell of your body. While you exhale, feel that you are getting rid of stale, poisonous air.

Ten breaths will suffice. Your suggestion will have taken shape.

I must point out that a suggestion is not necessarily logical. Logic is not a precondition for success. Success depends on the vividness and precision with which the mental image is implanted.

Any man who is capable of belief — and who of us is not — is by that capability suggestible. The infallible way to be effective is to repeat a clearly stated suggestion. But do not exceed three repetitions per session.

HOW TO OBTAIN WHAT YOU DESIRE

In every aspect of your life, success begins with mental images. The right image brings the right result. This law is unswervable.

Failures also come from accepted images. Example: There are many times where you identify with your faults, and repeat:

"I can't do it . . . That does not suit me . . . It's the way I am . . ."

By giving in to these negative thoughts, you will forge a negative personality for yourself.

Every negative thought must be immediately counteracted by a positive thought. In this way, you hypnotize yourself into a life of success and joy.

HOW TO IMMEDIATELY CHANGE THE WAY A PERSON'S BODY WORKS BY HYPNOSIS.

I'm going to give you a sample exercise which will prove the power of suggestion.

Hypnotize someone as shown below. Base your suggestions on feelings or impressions that person has already experienced. You will be able to obtain an acceleration of his pulse, low blood pressure, considerable perspiration and sobbing. Then, with no transition whatever, you will produce a burst of laughter and euphoria.

Other movements, independently of our will, are produced by suggestion: deeper breathing, easier bowel movements, painless childbirth and the suppression of insomnia.

HOW TO INCREASE THE EFFECT OF SUGGESTION

Several factors play a part:

1. Your own personality, which will be greatly strengthened by these volumes.

   ☐ The ascendancy exerted by your more powerful personality over the patient.

☐ Your spoken word. Its content shall be intelligible. Its tone shall be monotonous, gentle but firm.

☐ Your bearing and behavior as you are treating him. Behavior and gestures stimulate or reduce the effectiveness of the suggestion made.

2. The individuality of the patient.

☐ Adapt your suggestion to his ability to create a mental image of the idea given. Something that will have an impression on one person will have no effect on another. Test different phrasings of the same suggestion, until you reach one he will follow.

3. The content of the suggestion.

☐ Every command that goes against the patient's inclinations encounters resistance to its realization. This must therefore be avoided.

DIRECT OR INDIRECT SUGGESTIONS

The conscious self often rejects a direct suggestion. If indirect, it more easily avoids the censorship of reason, which is inclined to be critical. Thus, this indirect form of suggestion will be more readily accepted and followed.

Why? Because the subject is unaware that this is the first of a succession of suggestions that will gradually and gently cause him to follow your will.

Here is an example of indirect suggestion that works:

A child refuses to sleep without the aid of a sedative. Her mother offers a candy instead of the sedative pill and says:

"Take this tablet and you will sleep".

(This suggestion is indirect, because the mother implies that the tablet is a sedative, but does not say that it is. Nor, of course, does she say that the tablet is candy, and not a sedative)

The child believes she has swallowed a sedative. (This is an auto-suggestion — a command from the child's unconscious to her body, which follows from her mother's suggestion.) She falls asleep. This is the final effect.

And here is an example of a direct suggestion that does not work:

After a rough day, say to yourself:

"I will count up to three, then I will feel fresh and alert".

You will experience nothing. The subconscious will simply not be convinced. Why? Because you have given an outright command, instead of an indirect image that contains and disguises that command.

You have not followed the logic of the unconscious. You have tried to force it, instead of letting it follow the natural conclusion of the images you give it. It will therefore resist the direct suggestion, and you will achieve nothing.

HOW TO RESTATE DIRECT SUGGESTIONS SO THAT THEY BECOME VIVID, INDIRECT IMAGES

In the same situation, frame the suggestion in this way:

"I'm going to take a cold shower, then I will be fresh and alert".

This suggestion will be realized.

Why? Because, this way, you are giving a physical image, rather than an abstract command. You are not commanding, "Count down 1-2-3". Instead, you are giving your subconscious a gratifying sensual picture to follow.

Once the subconscious is given such a picture, it can build a chain of associations from there. It can feel the soothing water in the shower, for example. It can magnify the vigor that the chill of the water gives you. It can turn every drop of that water into a "fountain of youth" for you.

Your unconscious must have a physical image to begin with. It takes this physical image, and builds on it — automatically — again and again and again — to give you the final result you want.

This is the way to make it work for you!

Dr. Liek relates a similar example in his book, *Das Wunder in der Heilkunde*:

"At the age of ten, I had countless warts on my hands. During a stay in the country, the servant made for me a cure for my warts. She knotted a thread around each wart, let some water run over each, and buried the thread at the place where the rain fell to earth from the roof. 'When these threads have rotted, the warts will disappear', she said. Six weeks later, without having undergone any treatment, I had no more warts".

This example demonstrates the power of vivid, physical suggestion, started by an "if . . . then" chain.

Alas, most often we use this kind of suggestion in its negative form.

For example: "If I go to the theater this evening, then I will surely have my migraine".

Therefore, express only positive ones of this type:

"If I regularly take this medicine prescribed by the doctor, I will soon be cured".

DOUBT: THE WORST ENEMY

Most of the time, we "want" to believe but we "cannot". The obstacles that block us are fear and doubt.

Therefore, to achieve the result you want, make a choice between negative and positive thoughts. Remember Edison. He carried out three thousand experiments to get to the point of constructing a single electric bulb.

Three thousand tests! Three thousand failures! But positive suggestion prevailed because he put them in these terms:

"I will succeed no matter what the cost!"

Thus, through this means, he succeeded.

Here is a rule: Every positive suggestion which tries to take root in a skeptical person bounces off the trained indifference of his subconscious. Destroy this self-defeating habit. Believe, and it shall be given to you.

SELF-CONFIDENCE

Believe in your powers. Use the power of suggestion.
No doubt must remain.
You will change your life . . . permanently.

HERE ARE MORE CONFIRMING EXPERIMENTS

When phrased correctly, certain suggestions are realized right away. The experiments described in the works of Dr. Franz Volgyest, *Menchen Und Tierhypnose — Die Seele Ist Alles* (Ed. Orell-Fussli), provide the proof.

Here is one such experiment:

To execute an examination of the hypnotic effects on the stomach, he had made several patients swallow a small probe. Then these people were put under hypnosis. The probes were still in place. He suggested to them that they were swallowing various foods.

Here are the laboratory analysis results:

Gastric secretion had changed in quantity and quality according to the food suggested.

For example: The suggestion of a patient's favorite dish produced a considerable rush of gastric juice.

The physician then made the following remark:

"How good would it be if you had actually swallowed that favorite food?"

Immediately, the patient's stomach stopped all functioning, as if annoyed by the hoax. But the suggestion of other delights made it take up its work once more.

Here is another experiment:

Dr. Volgyesi suggested to a patient a total insensitiveness in one eye. An intern then gently thrust a needle into the connective tissue, which is normally painfully sensitive. The patient did not even blink the eye.

MORE ELEMENTS OF SUCCESSFUL SUGGESTION

Let us begin with the experiment of L. Benedek. He suggested to a woman, "I am pouring hot water over your arm". The temperature of her skin went up three degrees.

Here are the elements that make up such a successful suggestion:

- ☐ Conscious concentration is limited. The patient's attention is fixed on a single idea — the suggestion — that starts outside the field of his consciousness.

- ☐ Through that suggestion, the patient imagines that a physical or psychic event has happened or is about to happen.

Suggestion is the basis of all hypnotherapy. Its power is useful in suppressing an illness or in curing it by natural means.

Conclusion: Hypnosis can be effective where all other therapy has failed.

IS HYPNOSIS DANGEROUS?

Many of my colleagues maintain: "Hypnosis is dangerous". I object! I have carried out thousands of hypnoses. I have never been confronted by a truly dangerous situation. I will relate, in all sincerity, several incidents, or "breakdowns", that occurred at the beginning of my career.

HOW TO PREVENT ANY DANGER WHEN YOU PRACTICE HYPNOSIS

One day, I put an overly-curious female journalist under hypnosis. My suggestion was this:

"You have the mental age of three years".

My son was, at this time, of the same age. He understood quite quickly that although his "new aunt" was big . . . she was a child. He led her into his room.

I watched them play quietly together. I intervened only once. The journalist wanted to get into the tiny bed . . . ! Then she discovered the television set. Fascinated, she turned it on and off, changed the channels according to my son's instructions. Note that, in her childhood, television sets did not exist.

But here was the problem. I wanted to put an end to the hypnosis. But I had no effect. The patient, too long in the hypnotic state, was totally reliving her hypnotic role of being a child.

What was I to do? I remembered having learned that in case of a "breakdown", I must keep cool and — above all — I must deepen the hypnosis.

I placed my hands over the eyes of the journalist and pronounced the following deepening suggestions:

"Now we will learn mathematics. You will like mathematics. I will teach you to count up to three . . . On three, you will open your eyes . . . You will feel refreshed and alert . . . You are twenty-three years old . . . Everything will be as it was before we began . . . 1 - 2 - 3".

The patient opened her eyes, remembering nothing.

BLOCKAGE OF SELF-HYPNOSIS

Here is another incident. I had suggested to someone:

"You can practice self-hypnosis only in my presence. But entrust your commands to me".

No sooner said than done. I heard the patient say to himself:

"I'm counting to three . . . on three, I will fall asleep . . . No one will be able to reawaken me . . . 1 - 2 - 3".

In his ignorance, he had committed a huge error! The last part of his suggestion placed both of us in the position of being incapable of bringing the hypnosis to an end.

It was necessary to eliminate this "blockage" so he could escape the hypnotic state.

ANNIHILATING THE BLOCKAGE

I proceeded to make deepening suggestions:

"You are in a deep sleep . . . Very deep . . . No-one will reawaken you . . . No one else will awaken you. . . . Only you will awaken yourself . . . Now, you are awake . . . Open your eyes".

Which he did immediately. Why? Because I did not try to work against his suggestion. I did not try to deny his suggestion.

By insinuating that he awaken on his own initiative — that no one else but himself awaken him — I allowed his subconscious to carry out the command he had given it.

I did this by suggesting that he was different than the "no one" that could not awaken him. I expanded this "no one" until it became "no one else". Therefore, he could now awaken himself without coming into conflict with his suggestion that no one could awaken him.

To conclude: Never give a suggestion that is contrary to the preceding one. In case of "breakdown", deepen it instead. Work your way around it in words. Follow this advice and any possible breakdowns will be negligible and harmless.

OTHER EXAMPLES TO HELP YOU AVOID EMBARRASSING INCIDENTS

Dr. Frauz Volgiesi recounts a curious "breakdown". One day, a mother came to consult him with her daughter who was suffering from menstrual irregularities. Under hypnosis the daughter received the following suggestion:

"At noon on a given day your period will begin".

The mother had insisted on being present at the procedure. On the given day, menstruation appeared in the daughter and . . . in the mother!

Where is the danger? It is in the poorly formulated and unrepeated suggestions. What should have been said was this:

"At noon on a given day, you, (give the daughter's name), will have your period. Only you will have your period, and not your mother."

Here is a another classic experiment of how a beginner can go wrong in doing hypnosis:

A patient drinks a large glass of water. You suggest:

"You are drinking cognac".

He will then be in a really drunken state. But, before you leave him, you must say:

"You now realize that what you have just swallowed is not cognac, but water".

If, on the other hand, the suggestion is left incomplete — if you do not tell him before you bring him out of hypnosis that water is not cognac, then that person will become tipsy every time he drinks a glass of water.

AUTHORITIES ON THE SUBJECT HAVE THEIR SAY

Is hypnosis dangerous, harmful? Well-known hypnotherapists refute this hypothesis.

Dr. Liébeault, founder of hypnotherapy, writes:

"I have practiced hypnotherapy for many long years. I am therefore in a position to declare this: it far surpasses all medical treatment. Unlike the latter, it is without danger, without counter-indication and acts very quickly".

Dr. Brügelmann of Baderborn replies:

"To the question: a hypnosis carried out according to the rules of the art, is it dangerous? I reply with a categorical 'no' ".

Dr. Moll adds:

"To the question: suggestion under a hypnosis appropriately executed, is it a danger to health? I respond with an absolute 'no' ".

Dr. Ringuier of Zurich:

"I repeat what I have already stated: I have never detected a harmful influence during hypnotherapy".

Dr. Scholtz of Bremen says:

"I have never discovered dangerous consequences, neither during nor after an operation. These have been trumped up by our detractors, on the basis of false information".

Dr. Möbing states:

"Physicians warn against hypnotherapy. They are detractors of hypnotic suggestion. They base this solely on theoretical suppositions".

Dr. Otto Wetterstrand comments:

"I predict a great future for hypnotism. I am of Professor Bernheim's opinion. His remarkable work proves that hypnotherapy is one of the most precious possessions of present-day medicine".

And I add:

"The only existing danger arises from ignorance on the part of the therapist or of the amateur".

TECHNIQUES FOR QUESTIONING THE PATIENT'S SUBCONSCIOUS

THE CARPENTER EFFECT AND THE IDEOMOTIVE LAW.

In 1974, Dr. W.B. Carpenter discovered that "The IDEA of a movement engenders a lessened physical reaction to it". I will explain this in one moment.

The same year, he published a collection of his discoveries. The title of his book was *The Ideomotive Law*.

We apply this law in the following pendulum experiments. It is called "The Carpenter Effect".

Let us understand how this vital law works. Let us start with the mere IDEA of a movement — for example, the suggestion by someone else that you should walk across the room. In your normal waking state, this IDEA attempts to force itself on your consciousness.

But in your normal waking state, there is an obstacle . . . the critical faculty of your consciousness. In consequence, the field of your conscious possibility is limited. Therefore, you can accept only a weak realization of that idea. Therefore, you may or may not follow the suggestion and walk across the room.

But, under hypnosis, the mental IMAGE is beyond the control of your consciousness, and therefore tends to be accepted and acted upon. You are many, many times more likely to obey the suggestion, and walk across the room.

Therefore, in your own practice of hypnosis, it is vital to suggest ideas that are linked with vivid emotions and are transformable into images. And that, therefore, can escape the critical, blocking faculty of your consciousness.

THE PENDULUM EXPERIMENT

To prove the effectiveness of the Carpenter effects, I propose the following experiment:

Here is the procedure:

Trace a cross on a blank sheet of paper. Make a pendulum by suspending a ring on a thread 18 inches in length. The diameter, weight and material have no influence on the result.

Roll the thread around your index finger. Let about 8 inches remain between the ring and your finger.

Perform this experiment:

Hold the pendulum directly above the center of the cross at the intersection of the two arms. The pendulum is motionless. Your hand does not move.

Now make a mental image of the design. Concentrate harder. Concentrate still harder.

See the four sides of the cross. See them inside your mind, as well as on the table below you. See how they could be joined together by the pendulum. How it could travel, by itself, from one side of the cross to another.

The pendulum will soon make circles around the cross.

Stop its motion. Now, identify yourself more and more deeply with this mental image. Become the cross. Become the circle the ring had made around it.

Believe that the ring must make — should make — a circle around that cross.

Your idea will again become reality. The circular movements of the pendulum are now a concrete representation of your ideas.

We have just discovered The First Law.

FIRST LAW

Every mental image which asserts itself until it is believed tends to be realized.

What is the prime condition required for its realization? Never formulate an second idea opposed to the first.

If, for example, you suddenly believe that the pendulum should not circle the cross, then that new and contradictory belief is like a command to shut off your unconscious.

In this case, the pendulum will stop its circling, even though you have not consciously told it to stop. Your unconscious cannot hold together two opposing ideas.

So train your thoughts to run in one given direction only. The result will be guaranteed.

Eliminate doubt. It is an obstacle to the realization of the mental image.

Conviction — and conviction alone — produces the result. We have just discovered the second law.

SECOND LAW

If the conscious will and the unconscious conviction are opposed, the unconscious conviction will prevail.

Example: we do not "want" to move our hand but we "believe" in the movement of the pendulum. The anticipated movement will take place.

Our mental images, far deeper than our thoughts, control our lives. Let these positive images take root in your subconscious, which then becomes a submissive worker. You will then become master of your fate.

Do you envy individuals who succeed in their lives? These are their secrets:

They concentrate solely on the mental image of the desired goal.

They eliminate every defeatist idea that insinuates itself.

This is the principle of the third law.

THIRD LAW

All naive effort defeats itself.

To explain: A naive effort of will remains sterile in its effect. You will actually achieve the opposite of the result you desire.

As an example: You try to force yourself to stop smoking. After a short while, however, your will cracks and you find yourself smoking even more.

I repeat: Your thoughts forge your destiny.

Do not let them wander at the whim of your imagination.

Once mastered, they will be the positive elements of a very successful life.

WORKING OUT A CODE TO QUESTION YOUR UNCONSCIOUS

To use the pendulum experiments for this purpose, work out three movements: "yes", "no", "I don't know". Your subconscious will then choose one of these movements to tell you what you would otherwise never know.

Here is how it's done:

The pendulum is motionless. Think now:

"What movement will mean 'yes'?"

Observe the pendulum. It will slowly begin to move in one direction. This direction is therefore its code to you for "yes".

Restart the exercise to define "no".

Then start it again to define "I don't know".

HOW TO QUESTION YOUR UNCONSCIOUS

To do this correctly, ask only for "yes" or "no". How is this done? First, hold the pendulum motionless above the cross.

Ask your unconscious a question. For example, "Will I be a powerful hypnotist?"

Your subconscious will most probably reply, "yes". Then continue with your other questions.

This technique allows you to question your subconscious.

As a consequence you will learn to know yourself far better than ever before.

Every day, continue to train yourself in this self-revelation technique.

As an extra bonus, you will also be able to question your subconscious concerning your fellow man, whether he be present or absent.

A SECOND KEY TO THE UNCONSCIOUS: INVOLUNTARY MOVEMENTS OF YOUR FINGERS

This is another procedure which uses the Carpenter effect, and allows you to explore your subconscious by means of a very simple technique:

To do it, resume the preceding experiment. Define the "yesses" and "no's" with your fingers.

Example: involuntary movement of the index finger will mean "yes"; but involuntary movement of the middle finger will mean "no".

YOUR SUBCONSCIOUS DECIDES WHICH CODE TO USE

Let your subconscious decide it. Choose the method that suits you best, the pendulum or the movement of the fingers.

Here is how you induce the finger code. Place either hand on the table, fingers spread slightly. Now, wait for the finger's response.

THE FINGER'S RESPONSE

You feel a slight tingling or quivering. The finger more or less stiffens. Avoid all conscious effort: the finger will reply. Let yourself be surprised. Any "anticipation" will distort the result.

If you must make a decision, question your subconscious by means of one or the other of these two procedures.

RELAXATION USING THE YANG AND YIN

The universe rests in an equilibrium achieved by two opposing forces: tension and relaxation. In Chinese, these are named, Yang and Yin.

Man, an integral part of the cosmic harmony, attains his "ideal" state through relaxation. Harmony generates happiness and health. Let this equilibrium be broken and the human being will be disrupted. (Theory of Lao-Tse, 2500 years ago).

HOW TO ACHIEVE TRUE RELAXATION

True relaxation eliminates high tension, an obstacle on the road to happiness.

Its effect will be to put you in harmony with yourself and with the cosmic laws . . . to enable you to be in your best physical and psychic condition.   Also, relaxation eliminates illness, for illness is but an external sign of inner disharmony.

There are different methods: Autogenic Training, meditation, and prayer. But the most effective procedures are certainly hypnosis of others and self-hypnosis.

Hypnotic suggestion can bring about total relaxation.

In later volumes, I will give you the simple, automatic procedures.

Volume II

Master Secrets of Practicing Hypnosis On Others

EDITOR'S PREFACE

Here you are, ready to tackle the most important part of this course: putting patients under hypnosis, the different methods of doing so, the tests you must use, and the possibilities you have.

Remember that you have in your hands a truly professional, perfectly developed method. It is a Master who speaks to you. Everyday, he practices this art. Each method that he proposes, he has tested, checked, and perfected before proposing it to you.

The texts in *large italics* should preferably be learned by heart. Every word counts, and before you can compose your own formulas, you should be sure of knowing tested formulas which will protect you from the embarrassing silence of a lack of inspiration.

As in the manner of the great painters, begin by copying your master's work as perfectly as possible. Afterward, you will free yourself of the model and adopt your own style as you gain more practice in hypnosis.

In this volume you will learn the true language of the subconscious. You will discover the art of formulating suggestions in such a way that they obtain near miraculous effects.

The formidable power of the subconscious mind will be in your hands. Do not abuse your new powers. As Prof. Tepperwein comments, if you act only for your own profit without taking others into account, if you act without conscience ("Science without conscience is naught but ruin of the soul", said Rabelais), your subconscious will assume the implacable role of the judge. What you have gained by evil actions will be taken from you sooner or later.

There is a natural law of equilibrium between the forces of good and evil, between the powers of health and illness, between success and failure, between darkness and light. But you will learn to tilt this balance — to good, to health, to success — by hypnosis in this volume — and, in volume 4, by self-hypnosis.

Each of the methods of the great masters of hypnosis will be revealed to you in detail here. Dozens of closely-guarded, never-before-revealed secrets of hypnosis will be yours.

Prof. Tepperwein will tell you how he himself proceeds, what he says to his patients, how he develops the suggestions he will formulate under hypnosis, and in what manner he completely reassures his subject by removing all apprehension and hesitation.

This modern form of a session of hypnosis is more consistent with the spirit of holistic medicine . . . with the modern paths of the expansion of consciousness which liberate the individual, not enslave him.

By mastering the techniques of hypnosis, you will help your fellow man to set free whatever is most positive within himself. You also will benefit immeasurably, but this should not be your only goal.

The strength you will develop within you, the powers you will have at your disposal will not be gained at the expense of others. They are qualities for which you already possess the potential, and that you will gradually develop while putting your new talents at the service of others.

This volume is the most important: you should master it perfectly and avoid all "manipulation" of the subconscious of your subject. Let me remind you of the commitment that you made when obtaining this system:

"I pledge to use hypnosis only in the therapeutic spheres in which I am qualified."

"If I am not a qualified therapist, I pledge to use hypnosis only for purposes that are not of a medical nature, such as: correction of bad habits, learning improvement, development of memory and concentration, improvement of self-confidence and of assurance in public, training for sports, collaboration with the police for research, depositions, etc., everything that is not in the medical or therapeutic sphere.

"I pledge not to practice hypnosis on a minor, without the written agreement of his parents or his tutor.

"I also promise to respect the rights and wishes of my subject, and to always give him suggestions of well-being and harmony before awakening him.

"I attest that my desire to acquire your system is motivated solely by praiseworthy goals and that I will make use of my new knowledge only within the framework of the laws in force in my country . . . "

I wish you all success in your first experiments, and "may the Force be with you!"

Christian H. Godefroy,

Editor

UNDER WHAT CONDITIONS CAN HYPNOSIS BE PRACTICED?

HOW ARE ITS TECHNIQUES APPLIED?

PERSONALITIES OF THE HYPNOTIST AND THE PERSON TO BE HYPNOTIZED

DIFFERENT FORMS OF THE POWER OF SUGGESTION

My experiments have proved the following reality: every being is hypnotizable, and every person is a potential hypnotist.

Every individual possesses the power of suggestion to a greater or lesser degree. We make the distinction between psychically active natures and psychically passive natures. The psychically active individual impresses those around him. His principal characteristics are an obvious self-awareness and an unquenchable confidence. Such a person has all the qualities necessary to become a good hypnotist.

On the other hand, the psychically passive human being has little influence on those around him. A good hypnotic subject, he will also become a hypnotist — but only with effort.

It can therefore be stated that any intelligent individual, blessed with the ability and persistance necessary to develop a degree of confidence, and thus become sure of himself, undoubtedly possesses hypnotic talent. These require neither a mystic gift nor a penetrating gaze.

The conditions indispensable for permitting someone to rise above the norm are as obtainable as the following: a striking personality and the power to penetrate the mind of a stranger. Both depend on your willingness to develop your self-confidence.

As a result, all you have to do is develop your self-confidence.

Think of the old proverb: nobody believes in the one who does not believe in himself.

WHY MUST YOU CONVINCE WITH ENTHUSIASM?

The investigator A. Forel offers the following opinion: the best hypnotist is not necessarily the one who only *demonstates* to others his gifts. In this case, he will give them nothing more than some degree of *interest* in hypnosis. But only his personal enthusiasm will lead them to *believe* — and therefore to be hypnotized.

Therefore, to be utterly convincing, be utterly convinced yourself.

An entertainer's talents are, of course, not required. The best means of persuasion (for example, by giving the patient a transforming personal experience) leads through word-of-mouth to the so-called "contagious hypnosis".

This is mass suggestion — the kind of enthusiasm that overcomes all opposing opinions.

Suppose that the newspapers and television refer to you as an infallible hypnotist, capable of achieving hypnosis in a few seconds. Preceded by this type of publicity, you try to put some subjects into a hypnotic state.

You will succeed in all your experiments because your candidates, conditioned by excessive publicity, trusting and submissive, expect it to happen.

Now I will give you an example to the contrary.

If you approach someone and say, for instance, "I have never achieved a single hypnosis, I would like to try one last time," you will get no result because the candidate expects nothing of you. He will behave in a negative fashion.

YOU MUST EXPECT SUCCESS

True success for the hypnotist is not possible if he does not create beforehand the indispensable tension due to expectation. Only after that can he apply the mental image to be imposed.

It is therefore important to first gain the confidence of the person to be hypnotized, and to predispose him to put himself under your influence. This trust, linked to the hope of being able to believe in a result, conditions this positive attitude of expectation and leads to the creation of the correct mental images. In this state, success is assured.

Many people come to consult me, completely programmed for failure.

I often hear: "I have already been to three clinics. I have consulted many doctors. I have tried everything, to no avail. I am discouraged and in despair."

In such a case, I reeducate the person, teaching him to have confidence in himself. Only then do I begin to set the hypnosis in motion.

WHAT ARE THE QUALITIES YOU SHOULD DEVELOP IN YOURSELF?

Here are the qualities of the effective hypnotist:

☐ the gift of observation

☐ a taste for contact with others

☐ a great deal of patience

☐ presence of mind

☐ a pleasant voice

☐ a well-groomed appearance

☐ a striking personality

☐ the power to penetrate the mind of a stranger

☐ absolute confidence

This book will help you develop these qualities. The practice of hypnosis will give you an idea of your true personality. Instinctively, the patient will sense them. His behavior will be modelled on most of them.

HOW TO LEARN THE PATIENT'S
TRUE PERSONALITY

What is the patient's true personality? A dialogue will give you the answer. The very hypnosensitive people are the psychically passive, the unstable, and the drug addicts (really those on soft, prescription drugs). The latter are especially receptive to any suggestion and present a psychic condition parallel to the hypnotic state.

The absence of will is noticeable, as is the total inaction of the consciousness.

What are the conditions favorable to hypnosis? In the first place, the experience must take place without interuption. Therefore the surroundings play an important part. To avoid a negative physical reaction, soften the light in the room.

Let the patient notice these preparations. He will be only more ready to submit to hypnosis. Sometimes, however, too dark a room provokes fear. It's up to you to discover this.

Reflect well on the means to be used to trigger hypnosis. See if the subject is likely to submit to such an experience, and never lose sight of his well-being. If a procedure favors a rapid and deep hypnosis, if it does not harm the patient, its application is justified.

HAS THE PATIENT ALREADY BEEN HYPNOTIZED?

Has the patient already been hypnotized? By what means? These two questions must never be omitted. In general, a first hypnosis leaves traces behind. It would be preferable to adopt the same method that the last hypnotist used; the patient would prefer it.

Many people believe that suggestions are effective only under deep hypnosis. I advise you to correct this erroneous opinion. The patient must be persuaded that the depth of the hypnosis has no influence on the effectiveness of the suggestion.

In all cases, it is important to come up to the expectations of the subject being hypnotized for the first time. Try to induce a favorable state of mind and protect the person from any external stimuli.

MUSIC AND COLORS

Let the patient rest for a few moments, in a calm, softly lighted room. Soft music deepens this feeling of peace. The dominant colors of the decor contribute in no small measure to promoting this feeling of peaceful well-being. The right colors are green and blue.

You may replace the music by the ticking of a pendulum or a metronome. The monotony of this noise encourages drowsiness. But the most soothing effect by far is that produced by the sounds of the sea. Personally, I record them on an endless cassette. You can buy tapes on which special sounds are recorded.

FASTING

This is an excellent preparation for hypnosis. As everyone wants to lose weight, the patient will welcome your proposal to follow a diet. This will cause all resistance to subsequent methods applied to disappear.

TECHNIQUES REQUIRED FOR TRIGGERING A FIRST HYPNOSIS

You have a choice among numerous methods. I am going to help you to find yours and achieve a combination of several techniques.

First, some good advice:

Never say to your patient: "Now, I am starting to trigger the hypnosis". You will cause a tightening of the muscles and negative tension.

Say instead:

"I would like to know if you can relax. Start by lowering your arm".

Take hold of his arm and raise it slightly. Then, let go of it, and let it fall.

Resume the process with the other arm.

Now the patient must be reassured by telling him, for example:

"Everything will go very well ... Now, breathe calmly, regularly ... Close your eyes ... Nothing can distract you".

Next, you begin to put the hypnosis into effect. Here are some techniques.

TECHNIQUE NO. 1

THE PASSES OF MESMER

These hand passes are started two inches above the person. The movements are executed slowly from head to foot. Once you reach his feet, move back towards the head. Make these passes for five to ten minutes. The patient's eyes will eventually close.

Here are more details on how it's done. Begin making the passes at the head. Go slowly down to the feet while following a well-defined circular path.

From time to time, pass along the arms, over the chest, then go down once more to the feet. Now, go back up towards the head while making wide circles with your hands.

You will be amazed at the effectiveness of this method.

SPECIAL NOTE:

HOW CAN ANY HYPNOSIS BE STRENGTHENED BY MEANS OF CIRCULAR PASSES?

Here is how hypnotic passes in general are performed:

To begin with, hold your hands about two inches from the patient's head. You may also place them directly against his hair. Execute circular movements (as if you were washing the patient's hair).

Now proceed to the face area. Again, hold your hands about two inches from his face. Execute circular movements, as though you were drawing a halo around his head.

Now proceed to the chest area. Then the arms, the chest, the solar plexis, the genital area, the legs and the feet. Surround each area with circular halos, about two inches above the skin.

Then work your way back up again.

These gestures deepen the hypnotic state. They reinforce the patient's confidence in what you are doing for him. They intensify the power of the healing suggestions that accompany them.

TECHNIQUE NO. 2

FIXATION WITH THE INDEX FINGER

Hold your index finger eight inches above the patient's eyes. Tell him to watch it fixedly. His eyes tire quickly, then close. When they begin to blink, you can hasten their closing by giving the following command:

"Now close your eyes ... Your eyes are hermetically sealed ... You can no longer open them ... "

As a general rule, success is assured.

TECHNIQUE NO. 3

FIRST METHOD OF LEVITATION

This technique rests on an automatic movement of the fingers. Ask the patient to continuously stare at his hand. This type of passive self-fixation creates a strong tension due to anticipation and encourages the hoped-for movement. Say, for example:

"See, the index finger of your right hand is very gently beginning to rise. It is lighter and lighter ... Still lighter, lighter yet ... It is not rising any more ... "

From the first tremor of the finger, give the following suggestion:

"See, your index finger begins to move ... This movement grows noticeable ... More and more ... It becomes stronger and stronger ... More and more ... You are making no effort ... It

*rises by itself . . . Higher and higher . . .
Higher and higher".*

If the index finger rises, reinforce by the suggestion:

*"Feel it. The hypnosis is beginning to
take effect . . . Give yourself up more and
more to this pleasant feeling of weariness and heaviness . . . You feel more
and more tired . . . Nothing distracts
you . . . You are sinking still more into
this pleasant feeling . . . You are feeling
quite well".*

Suggest over and over to the patient:

*"You are quite well . . . Nothing distracts
you".*

TECHNIQUE NO. 4

SECOND METHOD OF LEVITATION

Give the patient, comfortably seated in an armchair,
the following suggestion:

*"Your arm is getting lighter and lighter.
Soon, it will begin to float . . . When it
touches your forehead, the hypnosis will
be deep".*

Repeat this suggestion and watch the patient carefully. I advise you to reinforce each of his movements by
means of an appropriate suggestion, like this:

*"You feel as if your fingers are becoming
lighter and lighter . . . Your fingers are
becoming lighter and lighter".*

Repeat these words until you obtain a slight shudder.
Reinforce:

*"See, your finger (the one that is quiver-
ing) is quite light and is beginning to
float. Soon, your whole hand will float!
Your hand will grow lighter and lighter
and begin to float. . .*

*"It rises higher and higher . . . Higher
and higher . . . As soon as your hand
touches your forehead, the hypnosis will
be deep . . . Feel it. Your hand rises
higher and higher . . . Now, it is touch-
ing your forehead . . . Feel it. Your
hypnosis is deep . . . You are deeply
under hypnosis . . . But, you hear
everything I tell you . . . You will obey all
my commands".*

TECHNIQUE NO. 5

PRESSURE OF THE ARM AGAINST THE WALL

The patient is told to stand against the wall, and lightly brush it with his forearm. This exerts pressure for thirty seconds. Then tell him to increase the pressure for the next ten seconds. Say:

"Your arm is quite flexible ... Now, it is beginning to rise automatically".

This rising of his arm is a natural consequence of any effort of this kind. This method will also give you an idea of the degree of susceptibility of the patient. The higher his arm rises, the more susceptible the patient.

TECHNIQUE NO. 6

RAISING THE ARM

The patient raises an arm and closes his eyes. Give him the following suggestion:

"You are sinking more and more deeply into a hypnotic state. Your hypnosis is becoming deeper and deeper ... Nothing distracts you ... You are sinking still further ... Into a hypnotic state ... The

deeper your hypnosis, the further your arm will fall . . . "

After five minutes have gone by, the arm will be lowered, the muscles relaxed. The pleasant feeling of heaviness he gains will be favorable to hypnosis. Deepen it with the help of these suggestions:

"Your arm is down . . . It is as heavy as lead . . . Your arm is relaxed . . . All the muscles of your body are loosening up . . . Now, they are quite relaxed . . . This pleasant relaxation is spreading through your body . . . Sit down comfortably . . . Now, I am leading you to a chair . . . Let yourself fall backwards . . . Feel it. Your hypnosis is becoming deeper and deeper . . . During your movement, your hypnosis is becoming deeper and deeper . . . Nothing is important anymore. Let this wonderful relaxation win over your body completely . . . Now, you are under deep hypnosis . . . Your subconscious is recording everything I say to you . . . You will obey my commands".

Give these suggestions to the patient. He will obey you.

TECHNIQUE NO. 7

SWIVELING

Place the patient in the center of the room. Ask him to close his eyes. Then gently take him by the shoulders and lean him backwards. Make sure he does not feel any fear of falling.

Lead him in circles either to the right or left. The patient will swivel completely around and will cross the room that way, following a figure eight. After a certain time, he will easily following you and will make perfect figue eights in the room.

Now, draw him towards a chair and make him sit down. The preceding movements have caused a slight dizziness, favorable for triggering the hypnosis. When hypnosis begins to show itself, deepen it with these words:

"Feel it. The hypnosis is beginning to take hold . . . Let yourself go . . . Let yourself fall, I am holding you . . . Nothing must distract you . . . You are sinking deeper and deeper . . . Now, you are seated comfortably . . . A pleasant feeling of relaxation is spreading throughout your body! Your hypnosis is becoming deeper still! Now, you are under deep hypnosis . . . Each one of my words is be-

ing established in your subconscious . . .
You will carry out my commands".

TECHNIQUE NO. 8

THE BLACK SPOT

The patient is lying comfortably on a couch. At the level of his eyes, attach a black spot, the size of a quarter, to the ceiling. The patient concentrates on this spot without blinking his eyes. Give him the suggestion:

"Feel it. You are keeping your eyes open
with difficulty . . . Your eyes grow heav-
ier and heavier . . . They will soon
close . . . Now, your eyes are very
heavy . . . You can hardly open them . . .
Feel it. Your eyes are closing . . . A won-
derful feeling of relaxation is spreading
through your body! You are surrender-
ing to this relaxation! Nothing can dis-
tract you any more . . . You feel light . . .
Free . . . You are relaxing more and
more . . . Nothing is important . . . Let
yourself go . . . Don't fight it . . . Let it
happen . . . You hear only my voice . . .
Your subconscious is recording all my
words. You will obey my commands".

TECHNIQUE NO. 9

HYPNOSIS UNDER HYPNOSIS

Once you become a past master of the techniques of hypnosis, you can attempt "hypnosis under hypnosis" in this way. First put yourself under hypnosis and deepen it by means of the appropriate techniques.

Then, give yourself the following suggestion:

"My hypnosis is deep . . . Nothing can distract me . . . But I can speak . . . While I speak, my hypnosis will become deeper still. At each of my words, it will become deeper and deeper".

Record these words on a cassette. In this state, hypnotize your patient. A mysterious fluid will emanate from your person. Hypnosis will be triggered very quickly in the subject to be treated.

TECHNIQUE NO. 10

THE YIN SYSTEM

The patient, lying on a couch, arms and legs limp, closes his eyes. Induce the yin from either the right or left side of the patient. It makes no difference whether you start on the left or right. Here is the way it's done:

Place yourself behind the patient. Put your hands on his head, then encircle it with your hands. Slide them from the head to the arms of the patient, passing by his shoulders. Now, put your hands around either his left or his right arm. Come down to his feet. Encircle his leg, then his foot, and go twelve inches beyond that.

Next, begin the operation again, starting from the other side of the head. Do not exert any pressure; let the weight of your hands do it. Repeat these movements eight times in a row on each side.

This technique produces in the patient perfect relaxation and deep sleep.

Transform this into hypnosis in these terms:

"Your peace is profound . . . Very profound . . . You can hear me . . . You hear distinctly everything I tell you . . . Your subconscious records each of my words . . . You will obey my commands . . . Raise your right hand!"

If the patient raises his hand, rapport will be established. In this case, you may give the desired suggestions. If he no longer reacts to your commands, blow into his face and repeat them.

This Chinese technique, with its profoundly soothing effect, can be integrated into any other method to trigger hypnosis.

TECHNIQUE NO. 11

COUNTING

With the patient seated or lying down, let him close his eyes. Give him the following suggestion:

"Soon, I will begin to count ... At each number, you will alternately open and close your eyes ... Slowly ... Calmly, from one number to another, your eyes will grow heavy ... You will open them with greater and greater difficulty ... Soon it will be impossible for you to open them ... Now, I am beginning to count ... At each number, you will open or close your eyes ... From one number to the next, your eyes will grow heavy ... One, your eyes are as heavy as lead ... Two, they are heavier and heavier ... Heavier and heavier ... Soon, you will not be able to open your eyes ... 3-4-5-6-7-8-9-10 ..."

If at the number ten, the patient still has his eyes open, begin again. Then, his eyes will remain closed even if you continue counting.

Deepen the hypnosis with these suggestions:

*"Now, your eyes are hermetically closed
and remain closed. You can open them
no more ... You no longer want to ...
You are surrendering completely to this
pleasant feeling of tiredness and heaviness ... You are more and more tired ...
More and more tired ... Your peace is
very profound ... You will obey all my
commands".*

TECHNIQUE NO. 12

COUNTING FROM 1 TO 10

This technique is effective if the patient is very suggestible. Lying comfortably, he closes his eyes. Give him
the following suggestion:

*"Put yourself at ease ... Nothing can
distract you ... You hear only my
words ... Apart from my words, nothing
is important any more ... You no longer
hear anything but my words ... I will
count slowly up to ten ... From one
number to another, you will sink more
and more deeply into a wonderful feeling of peace and relaxation ... At each
number, you will sink ever more*

*deeply ... At ten your peace will be pro-
found ... You will obey all my commands ... Now, I am beginning to
count ... One - two - three ... etc ... ten.
You can no longer open them ... Try ...
You will not succeed ... You can no
longer open your eyes ... You are no
longer trying to open them ... You are
giving yourself up more and more to this
wonderful feeling of peace and heaviness ... You hear everything I say ...
You will obey my commands".*

In case of failure, begin the procedure again at once.
As a general rule, success is assured.

TECHNIQUE NO. 13

COUNTING FROM 1 TO 100

The patient, lying or seated, closes his eyes. Say to
him:

*"Now, I will count slowly from one to a
hundred ... At each odd number, you
will open your eyes ... At each even
number, you will close them".*

Count quickly at first. Adapt the rhythm to the movements of the patient's eyes. He should not tire himself nor make any effort.

Progressively slow down the rhythm and suggest:

"From number to number, your eyes will grow heavy".

Now, do not count steadily any more. After each number, interpose a silence, so that his eyes will open briefly and close for a longer duration. Observe the patient: if he shows the slightest difficulty in opening his eyes, strengthen the suggestion in the following manner:

"Your eyelids are getting heavier and heavier . . . Soon you will no longer be able to open your eyes . . . Although I will continue to count, you will no longer be able to open your eyes . . . Your eyes are closing and remain closed . . . You will no longer be able to open your eyes . . . Your eyes are hermetically closed . . . A deep peace surrounds you".

TECHNIQUE NO. 14

STARING AT THE BASE OF THE NOSE

Place yourself in front of the seated patient. Tell him to watch the base of your nose or your right eye without blinking his eyes. Stare fixedly into both his eyes or one of them. Do not blink. Practice this effect fifteen minutes before the experiment. The patient's pupil will dilate, then contract. After some time, his sight will waver. Then give him the following suggestion:

"Soon, your sight will be blurred... The hypnosis will begin to take effect".

His pupil will dilate once more. Say:

"You see dimly... Slowly, you will sink deeper and deeper under hypnosis... Your eyes will grow heavier and heavier... Soon, they will close... Now, your eyes are so heavy that you can no longer keep them open... Your eyes are closing and remain closed... Feel it. A pleasant feeling of tiredness and heaviness envelops you... You will sink deeper and deeper into this wonderful feeling of fatigue and heaviness... You are more and more tired... More and more tired... "

TECHNIQUE NO. 15

SWALLOWING

Tell him, for instance:

"If you swallow your saliva several times in a row, I will deduce from that that the hypnosis has taken effect".

The patient will fix his attention on his swallowing. After a few minutes, he will do it the required several times, one right after another. Immediately reinforce the effect with the help of the following suggestions:

"Feel it. The hypnosis is beginning to take effect ... At each swallow, the hypnosis deepens ... This effect is growing, is enveloping you ... You are surrendering to it more and more .. Nothing can distract you any longer ... You will sink deeper and deeper into a pleasant feeling of tiredness and heaviness .. You are more and more tired ... More and more tired".

TECHNIQUE NO. 16

THE WARMTH OF THE HAND

The patient, lying on a couch, closes his eyes. Place your warm hand on his stomach. Give him the following suggestion:

"Feel it. A benevolent warmth emanates from my hand . . . A wonderful peace is spreading over your body . . . A certain well-being overcomes you, you are breathing slowly, regularly . . . At each breath you will sink deeper and deeper into this marvelous feeling of peace and safety. Nothing can distract you any more. This peace and this security cover you like a protective cloak . . . You are surrendering to it entirely . . . At each breath, you will sink deeper and deeper . . . Deeper and deeper . . . "

TECHNIQUE NO. 17

PILLS THAT TRIGGER HYPNOSIS

The patient rests for a moment. Before starting off hypnosis, administer one or two hypnotic pills — or placebos (a pill which contains no drugs, but which is hypnotic in its subjective effect: for example, one which is composed of lactose).

Tell him:

"These pills will take effect in a few minutes ... Surrender completely to this effect, detectable in the slow and regular rhythm of your breathing ... Your arms and legs will become heavy ... Your eyes will close".

Some patients will assure you that they have definitely felt the calming effect of the placebos. It met their expectations, encouraged by your suggestions.

This technique may be combined with others.

TECHNIQUE NO. 18

"THE FIST"

Place your hand on the table, then form a fist. Repeat this procedure with the other hand. Now, touch the region of the patient's heart with the fingertips of your right hand. Put the fingertips of your left hand on his forehead. These layings-on, combined with appropriate suggestions, will quickly produce a feeling of tiredness and heaviness. Convert it to hypnosis.

This technique may be allied with others.

TECHNIQUE NO. 19

FALLING

Stand behind the patient, standing in the middle of the room. Tell him:

"Soon you will fall backwards, but I will catch you. Be relaxed, look straight ahead. Surrender yourself... Prepare to submit to this force which will quickly manifest itself".

Place a hand on each side of the patient's head and tell him, for instance:

"Feel it. You are drawn irresistibly backwards... More and more..."

Withdraw your hands slowly and reinforce with the following suggestions:

"Now you are beginning to fall... You are falling backwards. You cannot prevent it... You are falling... Falling..."

A person who can be influenced will sway, then fall. Continue to speak:

"Now, you are falling... The force pushing you is uncoiling. You can no longer resist it... You are falling... I will

catch you . . . You are falling . . . You are falling . . . "

Repeat these suggestions until the patient falls into your arms. If he hesitates, command:

"Fall!"

Few will resist the influence of this technique.

Here is a supplementary trick to speed up the effect:

Stand beside the patient. Hold one hand twelve inches from his face; the other five centimeters behind his head.

Slowly bring your hand closer to his face, then order him to fall. By instinctively withdrawing your hand, the patient will throw his head back. This movement will help him to fall.

TECHNIQUE NO. 20

THE SUGGESTION OF HEAT

Gaze fixedly into the patient's eyes, as he is placed in front of you. He holds out his hand. Put a coin into it and suggest that this coin is getting warmer. Tell him:

"Feel it. The coin is getting warmer and warmer . . . Warmer and warmer . . . You clearly feel how it is heating up . . . Now

it is so hot, you can hardly hold it in your hand . . . It is becoming hotter and hotter . . . Hotter and hotter. You can no longer hold the coin in your hand. You must let it fall or you will burn yourself . . . Quickly, let it fall, you'll burn yourself . . . Let the coin fall".

Repeat these suggestions. The patient should eventually let go of the coin. But if he doesn't, add the following suggestion:

"See, you are not completely relaxed . . . Relax . . . Don't let yourself be distracted . . . Try again".

Then perform the experiment once more. You will succeed with 80% of your patients.

TECHNIQUE NO. 21

THE PENDULUM SUGGESTION

Put a pendulum into the patient's hand. You can make a pendulum by hanging a ring at the end of a length of thread. Weight and material have no bearing on the result. Say:

"The pendulum will swing as soon as the hypnosis begins to take effect".

Then reinforce with the following suggestions:

"You are calm ... Quite calm ... A wonderful peace is spreading through your body ... You are feeling very well ... A pleasant feeling of tiredness and heaviness pervades you. Surrender completely to this feeling ... Breathe slowly, regularly ... At each breath, you will sink more and more deeply into this feeling of calm and security ... The hypnosis is taking effect more and more. It is growing in strength and the pendulum is beginning to swing more and more ... Your hypnosis is deepening more and more ... Now, you are under deep hypnosis ... You will obey my commands ... You feel an absolute obligation to carry out my commands".

TECHNIQUE NO. 22

COUNTING BACKWARDS

The patient counts from a hundred to one. Unused to it, the conscious mind is occupied by the act of counting backwards.

During the counting, give the following suggestion:

"Your arms and legs are becoming heavier and heavier ... You will be more and more tired".

The conscious mind being occupied, your suggestion will easily reach the subconscious.

The patient will begin by counting distinctly, then his rhythm will slacken. The subject will omit numbers, then groups of numbers. From this signal, you will recognize the degree of effectiveness of your suggestions.

Repeat those which prove effective, then complete the triggering of the hypnosis in these terms:

"You are counting with greater and greater difficulty ... You are very tired and you would like to rest ... You can hardly speak ... You are surrendering more and more to this pleasant feeling of tiredness and heaviness ... Now, you can no longer talk ... Your hypnosis is deep ... Nothing can distract you anymore ... Nothing is important anymore ... Let yourself go. Let it come ... Let the effect happen ... You are listening to my words only ... They are registering in your subconscious ... You will obey my commands".

Make him follow the desired suggestions.

TECHNIQUE NO. 23

THE SUGGESTION OF THE ESCALATOR

Your patient rests for ten minutes.

During this time, he will concentrate, remaining calm and relaxed, on his slow and regular breathing. Eyes closed, he imagines himself at the top of an escalator, his hand on the rail.

Begin counting and suggest:

"Feel it. You are going down on the escalator . . . Each number represents a step . . . You are becoming more and more tired".

Try to discern any basic aversion to escalators. If there is none, begin to apply this very effective technique. The conscious mind, occupied with simulating this descent of an escalator, will pose no barrier to your suggestions, which will be registered in the patient's subconscious.

TECHNIQUE NO. 24

THE TOP OF THE HEAD AND THE EYEBROWS

The patient, seated before you, turns his back to you, and closes his eyes and concentrates on what you are about to do.

Begin with the head. Here is how you proceed:

Execute circular movements that do not quite touch the top of his head. Reinforce the mechanical effect with the help of appropriate suggestions, as I have given you before.

These movements, calm and regular, are done with the finger or the flat of the hand. The slight excitation thus obtained produces the expected effect.

Here is a variant of this technique.

The patient closes his eyes. Now make passes over his eyebrows. At the same time give the suggestion:

"Your eyelids are getting heavy . . . Soon you will no longer be able to open your eyes".

After five minutes, the patient will be incapable of opening them. The hypnosis has begun. Reinforce it with the help of appropriate suggestions.

TECHNIQUE NO. 25

HYPNOTIC OIL

This technique draws its inspiration from the celebrated "Placebo" effect. Obtain a small flask of oil with an odor that is strong but pleasant to smell. For instance, Chinese "medicinal" or Olbas oil. Assure the patient of the great hypnotic power of this oil.

Now, your candidate makes himself comfortable, closes his eyes, and concentrates on the coming hypnotic effect. Hold the open flask under his nose. He breathes deeply, regularly. Suggest at the same time:

"The hypnosis will be triggered after ten breaths".

Deepen the hypnosis by means of appropriate suggestions of peace. This technique may be combined with others.

TECHNIQUE NO. 26

IRRESISTIBLE FATIGUE

Here is a simple but effective technique, obtaining a result after ten minutes of application. It requires some confidence, both in the presentation and the subject matter.

Here is how it's done:

The patient is seated before you, in a highbacked armchair. He does not lean back in it. Instead, his back will be slightly inclined forward.

Here is his position you have him assume: His lower arms are held out in front of him. Then his upper arms come up straight, until they form a right angle. Then he closes his eyes.

Take hold of his hands and suggest to him that he feels irresistible fatigue. Lean against his hands and thus push him gently against the back of the chair.

Do not be surprised if your suggestion is already effective in some measure immediately. Every patient will complain of great tiredness and even of slight vertigo which the hypnosis will have encouraged.

This technique is also suitable for the practice of self-hypnosis. The following effect called "the barber's chair" or "the rocking chair" plays an important role here.

TECHNIQUE NO. 27

THE "BARBER'S CHAIR" OR "ROCKING CHAIR" EFFECT

The patient, seated before a mirror, watches his eyes unblinkingly. Place your left hand on his heart and your right on the nape of his neck. Begin with the suggestion of the heaviness of his eyes.

Reinforce the initial symptoms by means of appropriate words. If his eyes blink, give the command to close them, then rock the patient slowly backward. At the end of the experiment, he will of necessity be on his back. Now, deepen the hypnosis that has been triggered.

This type of action reinforces this "rocking chair effect".

TECHNIQUE NO. 28

THE BASE OF THE NOSE

With the eyes closed, the patient concentrates on the base of his nose. Now, execute passes by making slow, regular movements above his eyebrows. Begin on either the right or left side.

Give him the following suggestions:

"You are breathing slowly, regularly . . . You are feeling very well . . . At each exhalation, you surrender more to a feeling of tiredness and heaviness which overcomes you . . . Nothing can distract you . . . Nothing is important . . . You are surrendering completely to this feeling of tiredness and heaviness and you will sink deeper and deeper into it".

In most cases, the hypnosis rapidly takes effect.

TECHNIQUE NO. 29

READING

The patient reads a newspaper or a book, slowly, in a low voice. He reads a word every three seconds, stopping and restarting . . . The effort required will be well nigh unbearable for the conscious mind. After a few minutes, the subconscious will be receptive to all your words. You can give, for instance, the following suggestion:

"The hypnosis will begin after ten or twenty words".

This will happen in most cases. If your first effort does not succeed, you will need to repeat the procedure only once.

TECHNIQUE NO. 30

LAYING ON OF HANDS ON THE FOREHEAD AND THE NAPE OF THE NECK

Place one hand on the forehead, the index finger against the hairline. The other hand is to be placed on the nape of the neck, the index finger on the hairline. Deep breathing results from this, causing an objective and subjective hypnosis.

During this procedure, it is interesting to observe certain phenomena which occur under deep hypnosis. As long as your hands rest on the brow and back of the neck, the patient is unable to come out of the hypnotic state. The effect dissipates once the hands are removed.

This method of the laying on of hands, which triggers hypnosis by contact with the forehead and nape of the patient's neck, exceeds in strength the oral effectiveness of suggestion.

At one point, the patient's head seems to be enclosed in a vice, for this laying on of hands creates the feeling of a circle within the brain. You will achieve the same result if you withdraw your hands one or two inches from their former places.

Personally, I have interposed various objects between the patient's head and my hands. These in no way influence the proper progress of the procedure.

This remarkable technique is guaranteed to be effective at each application.

TECHNIQUE NO. 31

TENSING THE MUSCLES

The patient, lying comfortably on a couch, breathes slowly, regularly. While inhaling, he holds his breath for eight seconds and contracts his muscles. While exhaling, he relaxes the muscles of his body. The patient performs this exercise for ten minutes. This gives rise to great fatigue and a slowing of the heartbeat. Now, suggest to him:

"A feeling of tiredness and heaviness envelops you ... You are more and more tired ... Your breathing is slow, regular ... At each inhalation, you are surrendering to this feeling of tiredness and heaviness ... At each exhalation, you are sinking more and more into it ... You are feeling very well ... Your muscles are relaxed ... Feel it. Your arms and legs are as heavy as lead ... Your eyelids are getting heavier and heavier ... Now, they are very heavy ... You can no longer keep them open ... Now, you can no longer open your eyes ... They are hermetically closed ... You can no longer open them. You no longer want to open them ... You are more and more tired ... Everything I tell you is registered in your subconscious ... You will obey my commands".

This technique has always been successful for me.

TECHNIQUE NO. 32

A SPECIAL METHOD

This technique combines several methods.

I say to the patient lying comfortably on a couch:

"Raise your arms and legs twelve inches from the couch, for as long as you can".

Most patients lower their legs after thirty seconds. In this event, I command:

"Let your legs fall gently!"

I then command:

"After three minutes, you will let your arms fall! Your arms and legs remain relaxed on the couch".

His eyes closed, the patient relaxes for a minute. He breathes calmly, regularly. I then command:

"While inhaling, you will slightly lift your torso and legs and open your eyes. While exhaling, let your torso and legs fall and close your eyes".

This exercise produces a strong sensation of heaviness and relaxation. I deepen it with the help of the following suggestions:

"Now, your arms and legs are very heavy ... As heavy as lead ... They are getting heavier and heavier ... Feel it. This heaviness overcomes your arms and legs more and more ... Nothing is important any longer ... You are surrendering entirely to this feeling of heaviness and fatigue ... You are sinking into it still more ... Deeper and deeper ... Let yourself go ... Let it be ... Let the effect happen ... You are quite well ... Feel it. You are joyous, happy and free ... Your subsconscious is freed of all hindrance ... My words are being registered there ... You will obey my commands".

This technique guarantees you a result every time.

ACCESSORIES USED
TO TRIGGER HYPNOSIS

Little by little, each hypnotist develops his own method. For instance, take the patients of Dr. Wetterstrand. They gaze at the interior of a teaspoon, in which a candle flame is reflected. Other experimenters make them look directly at the flame. Yet others require the patient to contemplate his navel.

HYPNOSCOPES

Hypnoscopes have allowed the development of mechanical hypnotic procedures to take place. They combines the mechanical preparations which act on the patient's nervous system.

The simplest hypnoscopes are the pendulum of a clock and the regular tick-tock of a metronome.

Schupp has developed a "hypnoscopic" procedure, as follows:

Cover three square feet of a wall surface with black material. Place a metal disk at its center. Illuminate this with a projector. The patient will then concentrate on this luminous point and the hypnosis will take effect.

You may also use light bulbs of different colors or complicated geometric figures. Intense contemplation of them will fatigue the patient's eye muscles and he will close his eyes. A simple suggestion will suffice to deepen the hypnosis thus obtained.

THE STROBOSCOPE

This is a simple means of effecting a first hypnosis. However, it presents several difficulties. How is it done?

Make a hole in the centre of a mirror and hang it up. Make it revolve by some means. Now, project a beam of light upon the central hole of this mirror. The light will reflect various shapes in a steady rhythm. As a general rule the hypnosis will quickly take effect by this means.

You can also vary these devices so the dominant color changes in proportion to the mirror's speed of rotation — or to the speed at which the light is filtered.

For example, light reflected ten to twenty-times per second produces dominant colors that are reds and o-ranges. With a reflection of 13 and 14 times per second, you will get a green color. A rhythm of 15 to 16 times per second will produce a magnificent deep blue color. 18 re-flections per second gives a washed-out white.

(I should bring an important fact to your attention: a person suffering from latent epilepsy can suffer a crisis. The risk is not great — about one percent — but it exists.

DRUGS

All comments on the risks incurred by the absorption of drugs are superfluous. A great many people, the young in particular, have tried it. For centuries, hashish was used to cause hypnosis to take effect. Egypt, Syria and Persia made great use of it.

I will quote you an anecdote as an example.

The leaders of religious sects would promise their followers to show them paradise. Drugged with hashish, they were led into flowering gardens, where sensationally beautiful women overwhelmed them with voluptuousness and heavenly attentions.

Once out of the drugged state, the guru conditioned them in these terms:

"Blind obedience will be rewarded by eternity in this paradise!"

In this way, his followers would carry out his slightest command. They killed or caused to be killed in the hope of returning to this paradise.

HYPNOSIS CAUSED BY NARCOTICS

0. Wetterstrand and Krafft-Ebing quote cases of hypnoses effected with the aid of narcotics such as chloroform. Moll prefers chloral hydrate. Schupp uses ethylene

bromide. Narcotic palliatives are just as effective (Hallauer).

A. Friedlander describes in his book, *Die Hypnose und die Hypnonarkose (1920)*, the effect produced with the help of "Paradehyds" and several derivatives of barbiturates. The brief drunkeness caused by chlorethyline also encourages the hypnotic state.

I would note that to put hypnosis into effect by means of medication is reserved strictly for doctors.

FIXATION METHOD

This is the most ancient of the methods applied.

In Egypt, the priest-physicians held metal disks before their patients' eyes. The patients also gazed into clay cups with special patterns on them. These procedures made the eyes tired and produced hypnotic sleep.

EXTERNAL SIGNALS

Another effective means would be the inhalation of carbon dioxide in a mixture of three volumes of carbonic acid and seven volumes of oxygen. The inhalation of this mixture produces certain changes of the psychic faculty such as the ability to quickly catch impressions.

To explain: the strong concentration of carbonic acid in the blood reduces brain activity, hence inhibiting the reasoning faculty. The less this faculty is functioning, the more sensitive we are to "external signals".

COLOR CONTRAST METHOD

The method of Levy-Stuhl sets blue against yellow. The effects obtained are fatigue and personality change. They procure an advantage: sensory delusion, even among psychically active patients.

Here is the procedure:

Place a blue and then a yellow rectangle on a box. Separate them by a line one inch wide, and then test them yourself by looking steadily at the box for a few minutes.

You will obtain the following result:

On the yellow rectangle: the appearance of a light yellow line on the side placed against the blue rectangle.

On the blue rectangle: the appearance of a dark blue line on the side placed against the yellow rectangle.

Here is the experiment carried out by Levy-Stuhl and by Stockvis.

They gave these boxes to their patients. The patients looked steadily at the boxes. When they said that the color had changed, the experimenters suggested:

"You are under hypnosis".

This was deepened by the appropriate suggestions.

COMBINATION OF DIFFERENT TECHNIQUES

The hypnotherapist H. Scharl was inspired by the method of color contrast to improve it.

Here is Scharl's experiment:

Take a fairly large piece of cardboard, to the middle of which you glue a rectangle of dull red cloth. Mark the center of the cloth with a little black dot. On the white cardboard, paint another black dot directly below the first.

With the patient lying down, hold up his right hand. Place the cardboard with the red rectangle in that hand. He stares fixedly at the black dot within it.

Say this:

"Soon, a luminous border of a pale green color will take shape around the red surface. Your hypnosis is about to begin.

"Look at the black dot on the white cardboard ... Without blinking ... A luminous rectangle of a pale green color will appear ... Look at the black dot on the red cardboard ... Feel it. Your eyes are getting tired ... They want to close ... Do not resist ... Let your eyes close ... Lower the arm holding the cardboard".

EXPERIENCE IS THE BEST EXAMPLE

The surest way to effect hypnosis remains actual experience. Begin by selecting a highly suggestible person. He will easily fall under hypnosis and will serve as an example to other candidates who are more or less sensitive to hypnosis.

The trust and conviction of your patients will guarantee you a conclusive result.

DISTINCTIVE SIGNS OF HYPNOSIS

DEPTH OF THE HYPNOSIS

Many people confuse trance with hypnosis. In their minds, hypnosis implies total unconsciousness, where alien faculties can be introduced into the personalities of the patients.

But a large percentage of hypnosis is achieved from a medium depth of entry into the unconscious. This is enough to allow effective suggestions.

WHAT ARE THE DIFFERENT DEGREES OF DEPTH?

We recognize three degrees:

Light hypnosis: This is a state of relaxation during which the conscious mind remains active.

Medium hypnosis: This is a reinforced relaxation. Now the conscious mind is only marginally active. All suggestions in accord with the fundamental tendencies of the personality will be carried out. Also, when the patient returns to the waking state, he will obey posthypnotic commands.

Deep hypnosis: This is a state of absolute relaxation. The conscious mind is completely inactive. The patient will carry out illogical delayed suggestions. Upon awakening, the person remembers nothing.

To achieve a perfect hypnosis, you must follow the three degrees in succession, which will follow the order given above.

THE SIX DEGREES OF LIÉBEAULT

A. A. Liébeault recognizes six degrees:

1. Somnolence: The patient's eyes are heavy. He can no longer open his eyes. The conscious mind is wholly inactive.

2. Levitation: Perform a check by raising the patient's arm for a moment. Then lower it slowly. The fingers are flexible, the eyelids closed, the arms and legs not heavy. The conscious mind and the memory are functioning.

3. Rotational movements of the arms: The patient's sensitivity is clearly diminished. At this degree, the characteristics of the second degree are observed. Patients claim, "I did not act under hypnosis; I simply obeyed the suggestions given by the hypnotist".

4. The one hypnotized is dependent on the hypnotist: The patient no longer reacts to influences besides those of the hypnotist. At this stage, characteristics of the third degree are encountered.

5. Light somnambulism: The patient's sensitivity is either diminished or quite inexistent. You can suggest hallucinations. The conscious mind is disturbed and the memory proves defective. The "memory gaps" phenomenon is noticeable. At this stage, fourth degree characteristics are encountered.

6. Deep somnambulism: At this stage, certain fifth degree characteristics, reinforced, come into play. The conscious mind is not functioning at all. Reawakened, the patient will not remember any deed or action performed under hypnosis.

THE THIRTY GRADES OF DAVIS AND HUSBAND

Davis and Husband have established the following subdivision: (It is a classification of the symptoms of hypnosis into thirty degrees).

Putting under hypnosis:

1. Preparation for relaxation

2. Relaxation

3. Fluttering of the eyelids

4. Closing the eyes

5. Complete physical relaxation

Light trance:

6. Catalepsy of the eyelids

7. Catalepsy of the limbs

8. Stimulation of the effect

9. Stimulation of the effect

10. Cataleptic stiffness

11. Anesthesia (the gloved hand)

Medium trance:

12. Stimulation

13. Partial amnesia

14. Stimulation

15. Post-hypnotic anesthesia

16. Stimulation

17. Personality change

18. Simple post-hypnotic suggestions

19. Stimulation

20. Kinesthetic illusions and total amnesia

Deep trance:

21. The possibility of opening the eyes without reducing the depth of the trance

22. Stimulation

23. Receptivity to illogical post-hypnotic suggestions

24. Stimulation

25. Full somnambulism

26. Optical illusion of the senses, positive and posthypnotic

27. Auditive illusion of the senses, posthypnotic

28. Systematic posthypnotic amnesia

29. Auditive illusion of the senses, negative

30. Optical illusion of the senses, negative. Hyperesthesia

DOUBTS THAT MAY BE EXPRESSED TO YOU CONCERNING THE HYPNOTIC STATE

You may want to have an answer to the following questions:

Does the patient carry out your suggestions in all respects? Does he also obey under light hypnosis?

An actual experiment will give you all the documentation you need to answer this question.

An American specialist in the subject states: "The hypnotic state does not exist". He hypnotized two groups of students at the University of Pennsylvania. Here is how he went about it:

With one of the groups, he brought forward hypnotized subjects whose right hands were motionless. He stated to the group that this lack of mobility was suited to hypnosis. He made a demonstration of hypnosis to the second group, but this time, he did not mention the hands. Then the two groups hypnotized each other. The student "hypnotists" knew nothing of the experience of those being hypnotized, and vice-versa.

The result: the participants of the first group held their right hands motionless; those of the second group did not.

Our answer to this is simple. We may conclude from this test that the patient allows himself to be hypnotized according to his convictions. We have already said this several times before.

For this reason, it is important to find the most appropriate suggestions before triggering a hypnosis.

THE SIX PHASES OF HYPNOSIS

PHASE 1: PREPARATION

To succeed, begin by giving the patient a favorable opinion of hypnosis. Eliminate all negative ideas. The room in which the experiment will take place will preferably be quiet, somewhat in shadow. The room temperature should be pleasant and conducive to well-being. The patient, lying comfortably, eyes closed, breathes slowly, regularly. He is perfectly relaxed.

What behavior should you adopt? You yourself are a model of serenity and masterfulness. Utter your words in a slow, monotone voice. They will be reassuring.

PHASE 2: CONCENTRATION

The patient of necessity withdraws from all stimulation coming from an external source. Relaxed and passive, he concentrates on the coming event. While watching a given point, he listens to your words only.

PHASE 3: RELAXATION

Here are the appropriate suggestions:

"You are quite calm ... Nothing is important anymore ... You no longer hear anything but my voice. Your arms and legs are flexible ... You are breathing calmly, regularly ... At each breath, you surrender more and more deeply to the pleasant feeling of tiredness and heaviness ... Let yourself go ... Let it be ... Let it happen ... Your thoughts are becoming fluid ... You feel extremely well".

These suggestions are to be repeated if necessary. It is essential to obtain complete relaxation of the patient in this phase.

PHASE 4: THE OBJECTIVE

In this phase, the goal which motivated the hypnosis is attained. The required suggestions are these:

"You are feeling free ... Relaxed ... Nothing can distract you ... You hear only my voice ... You will carry out to the letter everything I will now tell you ... Each of my words is registering in your subconscious ... You will obey my commands ... You cannot, nor do

you want, to act in any other way . . .
You will obey".

Now, ensure that the goals which brought the patient to you are followed.

PHASE 5: THE DEEPENING PROCESS

Every suggestion previously given will be reinforced and repeated. Try different formulas. For example:

"Feel it. The effect is taking place . . .
You clearly feel the way this beneficial
effect overcomes you more and more . . .
How it grows more and more . . . Day by
day . . . Day by day, everything is getting
better for you, in every way".

PHASE 6: ENDING THE HYPNOSIS

Reverse all suggestions with the exception of the most important: that which motivated the hypnosis. Give suggestions contrary to the preceding ones:

"Feel it. Strength is coming back to your
body. Your arms and legs are once more
flexible and capable of movement . . .
They are moving now . . . You are brim-

ming with strength and energy ... I will count up to three ... At three, you will open your eyes and you will be completely awake, full of energy ... One ... Two ... Three .. "

Once out of hypnosis, converse with the patient for a moment. This dialogue will allow you to discover any remnants which are still worrying the patient. These can thus be avoided or corrected during a second hypnosis.

A FINAL AND VERY USEFUL PIECE OF ADVICE

Upon greeting someone, you can get an idea of his degree of suggestibility. A simple handshake will be enough.

As a general rule, you will observe that dry hands denote a psychically active individual who is difficult to hypnotize. Damp hands are characteristic of a psychically passive person who falls quickly into a hypnotic state.

There are, of course, exceptions to the rule.

HOW TO INITIATE
A CONSULTATION

PREPARATORY DIALOGUE

It is necessary to converse with the patient so as to establish contact, to create an atmosphere of trust and sympathy. It is also a prime necessity to eliminate all incorrect conceptions of hypnosis, and all fears. Do not forget to mention this key phrase:

"Hypnosis is a natural phenomenon and is not to be confused with magic".

The expectation thus created will make success more likely.

WHAT IS RAPPORT?

It is the fact that the preparation we have described above will cause the conscious mind of the subject to be drawn closer to you, the hypnotist. This contact, called "rapport" reduces the critical faculty of the person, but some opposition always exists.

To quote an example: give a command that is contrary to the fundamental tendencies of the patient's personality and the hypnotic state will be automatically dissolved. This command was not in accord with the patient's wishes.

For example, present the hypnosis in these terms:

"In the course of our lives, we are often under hypnosis; upon waking in the morning, or while gazing distractedly at nothing. Therefore, there is no reason to be uneasy, for certainly nothing unusual will take place here".

Next, positive and negative traces from previous hypnosis must be taken into consideration. To do this, ask the following questions:

"Why did you seek me out?"

"Have you been hypnotized before?"

This last question is very important. A previous hypnosis always leaves positive or negative traces.

If you detect a positive trace. . . if the previous hypnosis was successful . . . then use the same technique to trigger your hypnosis (even if it does not suit you).

In the case of a negative trace, try to find the method previously used and avoid it.

Certain patients will come to you, confusing hypnosis with narcosis — or they will imagine that it causes a deep sleep followed by total unconsciousness. Therefore, convince the patient that this conviction is completely mistaken — that, under hypnosis, he can hear everything.

NOW INCREASE THE RAPPORT EVEN MORE

Now, be sure to define the hypnotic state as "a wonderful state of peace". Tell the patient:

"Hypnosis is a wonderful state of peace. Do not be afraid to reveal any secrets. Only questions you choose will be explored during our discussion. You will not touch on any other subject under hypnosis".

The patient will put to you the following question:

"Am I sure to wake up from the hypnosis?"

Dismiss these anxieties with a categorical "yes". Tell him that even if you should die of a heart attack on the spot, his reawakening would be assured. The hypnosis would then automatically be transformed into sleep and he would reawaken after having slept his fill.

Remember always — and share with your patient — that a properly executed hypnosis presents no danger at all to the patient.

To avoid any deception, try to determine what the patient wants as a result of it. But know that a single hypnotic session will not be enough to correct a fault of character, or to change a depressed individual into a model of optimism and the enjoyment of life.

Permit me to bring the following fact to your attention: the practice of hypnotherapy is reserved exclusively to physicians, and to health practitioners such as you are learning here to be. This personality transformation is not to be tried by the untrained amateur.

One last piece of advice: if the patient insists on the presence of a third person, accommodate this wish. Certain people are shy or inhibited in the absence of someone dear to them.

TRUE RELAXATION

The effects of relaxation are: becoming free of tension, suppressing the negative activity of hypertension, and re-establishing psychic equilibrium.

Relaxation is therefore a powerful means of attaining happiness and health.

Therefore, be in harmony with yourself and hypnosis will work miracles.

THE THREE LAWS OF HYPNOSIS

I explain them to my patients this way:

☐ First law: Any persistent mental image tends to become reality.

☐ Second law: If will and conviction are opposed, conviction will prevail.

☐ Third law: Any effort made under hypnosis produces an effect contrary to expectation.

AN OUTLINE OF AN EXAMPLE OF PREPARATORY DIALOGUE

These should be your opening statements.

"I am happy to meet you."

"Have you ever undergone hypnotherapy?"

"How long ago was this?"

"How was it done? Tell me its steps."

"What exactly do you expect of me if the hypnosis is successful?"

Now, establish trust by saying this:

"Under hypnosis, you will neither be in a trance nor will you be unconscious. You will hear everything that is going on around you.

"Once I reawaken you, you will remember everything in detail. I will not ask you any indiscreet questions. You will reveal no secrets.

"You and I will formulate helpful suggestions together, and it will be these that I will give you. You will always reawaken, even if I should drop dead during the session.

"Do you want a third person present?"

"The session will be recorded on a cassette which you will take away with you".

"Do you have any questions?"

"Let us begin".

"Seat yourself comfortably. Close your eyes. Concentrate on some happy event of your childhood. Create a very clear mental image of it and review the un-

folding of the event in detail. Immerse yourself in the atmosphere of the time period. In a few minutes, we will begin to induce hypnosis".

INTELLIGENCE AND WILL POWER ARE NO OBSTACLES

On the contrary, people of average intelligence who are weak-willed are difficult to hypnotize.

A "duel" between your will and the patient's simply does not take place. The will of the patient puts itself automatically at your service.

In fact, the patient's ability to concentrate allows hypnosis to take place. Intelligence and will combine to achieve this.

Are there any side effects?

There are no side effects to be feared, for hypnosis carried out according to the rules of the art presents no danger whatsover.

THE LANGUAGE OF THE SUBCONSCIOUS

Tell the patient:

"Submit passively to my commands, and create a mental image of what they contain. Let it all unfold like a movie".

To summarize: The image and the idea are the language of the subconscious. Therefore, formulate in your mind a precise idea of images that you want the patient to follow.

Tell him to be passive and not to reason things out. Remind him that all conscious thought is an obstacle. If conscious thought dominates, the suggestion will not reach his subconscious.

It is also necessary to present him with mental images that spontaneously arise in your mind as you treat him, but that are, of course, always oriented towards the goal to be attained.

THE DIFFERENT PHASES

Once again — and this degree of review is absolutely necessary — here are the phases I have found most successful:

☐ First phase — Preparation. I eliminate any incorrect ideas of hypnosis. I establish contact between the patient and myself. He turns his attention to my words.

☐ Second phase — Concentration. I do not let the patient be distracted. Nor do I let him distract himself.

☐ Third phase — Relaxation. I encourage the patient to let go, to let himself be carried along. I state that my words are beginning to have their effect.

☐ Fourth phase — Suggestion. I provide the flow of suggestions. They will be transformed by his unconscious into mental images. I then strengthen each suggestion.

☐ Fifth phase — Effect. I repeat the suggestions in other words. This strengthens their effect.

☐ Sixth phase — Ending the hypnosis. I awaken the patient with appropriate suggestions.

THE POINT OF FIXATION

Now let us run through a beginning hypnosis, after the opening remarks are finished.

For example: Ask him to concentrate on the shiny tip of a pen, a glass ball, a shiny button, or any other object. His eyes tire, then close. You may also use a hypnoscope or a stromboscope.

Here is a trick: Set a lamp behind the patient. Project the beam of light on the object. The effect will be strengthened.

Do place this point of fixation eight inches above the patient's line of sight. He will look at it sideways and upwards, and his eyes will quickly become tired.

Another secret: I have used a blue bulb as the point of fixation. The patient concentrates on the blue, a restful color.

Strengthen the effect with the following suggestions:

"Concentrate on the point of fixation . . . Without blinking . . Nothing distracts you . . . Look at the point . . . Nothing else is important . . . Feel it. Your eyes are smarting . . . More and more . . . They can hardly stay open . . . Your eyelids are drooping . . . Your eyelids are getting heavier . . . More and more . . . More and more often, your eyes are closing . . . Now, your eyes are closing . . . And remain closed".

HOW DO YOU GET HIS EYES TO CLOSE?

"Now, your eyes are closed ... Hermetically closed ... You can no longer open them ... You try ... You can't do it. You no longer try to open them ... You are sinking further and further ... Feel this marvelous feeling of peace and relaxation ... You are sinking still more, more and more ..."

The method of fixation, very ancient, is still used today. It is a basis for most of the preparatory techniques.

TRY IT YOURSELF

Seat yourself in a comfortable armchair. Close your eyes. Look upwards for one to two minutes. Now, try to open your eyes. You will find that your eyelids appear to be glued.

OR TRY THE FASCINATION METHOD

This is the classic and most widely-known procedure.

It is the hypnotic procedure that most patients will expect when they come to you. It merely consists of gazing directly into the eyes of the patient, which then brings about the hypnosis.

When you use it, therefore, you are acting exactly as the patient expects you to act. Because he already thinks that this is the way he can be hypnotized, he is all the more likely to slip into deep hypnosis as a result of it.

To establish this deep contact, simply look directly into his eyes. But first, set the stage in this way:

THE IDEAL POSITION

First position: The patient and you are facing each other, his knees between yours, and your hands on his knees or his shoulder.

Second position: He is lying down, and you are seated by his side, but slightly behind him. Now say this:

"I am sitting near the top of your head, behind you. Look at me without blinking ... Into one eye ... Always into the same eye. The hypnosis is begining ... You will see my eye distinctly, then indistinctly ... Your eyes are smarting ... They are becoming tired ... You try to open them ... With each effort, your eyes grow heavy ... And close ... You are sinking into a state of peace and relaxation".

HOW DO YOU CREATE THE TENSION OF EXPECTATION?

It is important to announce to him the state you hope to achieve by appropriate suggestions. These will create the tension of expectation, dissipated little by little by the hypnosis.

For example: He is lying down, and you are seated at his side. You sit so your face is about twelve inches above his. The latter's line of sight is superimposed on the hairline of the hypnotist.

Suggestions:

"You are lying comfortably . . . Breathe calmly, regularly . . . Look closely into my eyes . . . Nothing distracts you . . . Listen to my voice . . . Nothing is important . . . Listen to my voice".

"BLINKER" EFFECT

Place your hands near one side of his head. They thus come between the light and his head, protecting it like "blinkers". This procedure, called "the blinker effect", encourages contact and avoids all distractions.

Now observe the pupil of his eye and adapt your suggestions to its reactions.

Dilated pupil: reduced vision. He is begining to slip into hypnosis.

Normal pupil: very clear vision. The hypnosis has not yet taken effect.

In either case, say this:

"You are not focusing very clearly . . . The hypnosis is beginning . . . Feel it. Your eyes want to close . . . They are tiring . . . More and more . . . Your eyelids are getting so heavy . . . More and more".

At the moment his eyes close, say:

"Your eyes are closed . . . They will remain closed".

Put your thumbs on his eyelids and strengthen the hypnosis.

When his eyes close, gently put your thumbs on his eyelids to prevent them from trembling. This gives him a feeling of safety, which encourages the hypnosis.

Scharl slides his hand from the patient's forehead over his eyes. He leaves it there for a minute.

Follow up with deepening suggestions.

DEEPENING SUGGESTIONS

"Your eyes are completely closed . . . You are quite calm . . . You are sinking into a pleasant hypnotic state . . . You are hearing my voice . . . Nothing is important . . . Nothing distracts you . . . Feel it. Your head is growing heavy . . . More and more."

Increase the pressure of your hand on his forehead. Strengthen the feeling of heaviness of his head. Follow up with deepening suggestions.

You are now ready to begin any of the methods of hypnosis I have given you above.

RAPID HYPNOSIS — THE MOST ANCIENT OF METHODS

Now that you have been shown various procedures, try a few rapid methods.

In 1813, the abbot Faria, having travelled from Goa to live in Paris, instituted the most ancient method, that of the famous sleep!.

Here is how he went about it. He came quite close to the patient, stared fixedly into his eyes for several seconds. Suddenly he commanded, "Sleep".

About 50% of the candidates fell into a hypnotic state.

Note that his forceful personality, allied to his fame, considerably aided his success.

As you become more advanced, try this experiment. Put several people successfully under hypnosis. They will then provide publicity as your witnesses.

Now try it on other subjects. Already conditioned, they will surrender completely to your action.

THE AMERICAN METHOD

Test a prospective patient for his susceptibility to instant hypnosis.

How is it done? Place yourself in front of the patient, a little to one side. Put your left hand on his right shoulder. Form a "V" with the index and middle fingers of your right hand. Hold this figure at a distance of about twelve inches in front of the person's eyes.

Now suggest:

"Your eyes are growing heavier and heavier".

At the same time, bring the "V" up to his eyes. As soon as your fingers touch them from very close up, suggest:

*"Now, you can no longer keep your eyes
open . . . Your eyes are closing".*

Most people will close their eyes. Instinctively, the patient will try to avoid your fingers. This reflex will accelerate the effect.

If necessary, give the following command:

"Now close your eyes".

Put your hand on the subject's forehead, then slide it over his eyes. Follow up with appropriate suggestions to deepen the hypnosis obtained.

ANOTHER INSTANT METHOD: COUNTING

As a general rule, I obtain a most rapid result this way. I place the patient anywhere in the room. I suggest:

*"Soon, I will count from one to ten . . .
From one number to the next, your eyes
will grow heavy . . . More and more . . .
At the number ten, you will close your
eyes . . . When I have finished counting,
your eyes will be hermetically closed".*

I begin counting:

*"One, your eyelids are getting heavy . . .
Two, they are getting heavier and heav-*

*ier ... Three, they are as heavy as
lead ... Four, you can hardly keep your
eyes open ... Five, feel it ... Your eyes
want to close ... Six, they are closing ...
Now, you can no longer open them ...
Seven, your eyes are very heavy ... You
want to close them ... Eight, your eyes
are closing ... Nine, your eyes are
closing and remain closed ... Ten, they
are hermetically closed ... You can no
longer open them ... You no longer want
to. You are sinking more and more
deeply into this pleasant feeling of
heaviness and tiredness ... Feel it. It
pervades your whole body ... Your
subconscious is registering everything I
tell you ... You will obey ... My words
are taking root more and more in your
subconscious ... You will carry them out
to the letter".*

I then issue my suggestions.

This method allows hypnosis to be induced in twenty to thirty seconds. I obtain a success rate of 50%.

METHODS OF THE MASTERS

MESMER

The Schwabian doctor, A. Mesmer, introduced a certain form of hypnotherapy into France. He studied the theories of the celebrated physician of the time, Theophraste Bombast, called Paracelsus — as well as those of the Renaissance philosopher, Aggrippa von Nettesheim. The doctrine of animal magnetism is a combination of these theories.

According to Mesmer, someone's "magnetic force" can be transferred to another by the technique of passes executed according to well-defined designs.

This doctrine of the "Magnetic animal fluid" was first discounted, scorned and declared unscientific. However, the phenomena discovered by Mesmer were recognized by different magnetists. They contributed to the acceptance of hypnosis as a scientific fact.

These "passes" are called "mesmeric". The method of passes is called "mesmerism". Here is how it's done.

The patient is lying down. You begin your circular passes around his head, and descend to his feet along the arms and torso. These manipulations are carried out at a distance of two inches from the body.

Variant: you may exert slight pressure on those parts of the body mentioned above. Duration of treatment: ten minutes maximum.

When you feel he is ready, lift one of his arms. The arm should remain in this position.

In case of failure, repeat the passes for five more minutes.

The patient is now receptive to suggestion.

JAMES BRAID

The ophthalmologist James Braid made his discovery of hypnosis in 1841. He was present at a performance of hypnotic phenomena produced by the magnetist La Fontaine in Manchester.

Skeptical, he studied them with the sole object of denouncing this imposter.

His wife, his friend Walker and one of his domestic staff served as "guinea pigs". He held a shiny button for a moment at the level of the bridges of their noses. To his great astonishment, all three sank into a deep hypnotic sleep.

Braid had chosen this procedure by drawing on his professional experience. He knew that concentration of the eyes on a shiny object induced sleep from nervous fatigue.

He attributed the hypnotic effect not to the passes of the hand, but to the patient's imagination. Braid put his imprint on hypnosis. His fixation method, the basis of most techniques used to bring it about, is still widely used today.

Here is how it's done:

Hold a shiny object slightly above the patient's eyes. The eyes tire more quickly if the gaze is kept upward. Slowly bring your fingers towards the subject's eyes. They will begin to blink, then close.

In case of failure, repeat the experiment. Command:

"Feel it. Your eyes want to close. Close your eyes!"

Braid named the phenomenon "hypnosis", from the Greek name "Hypnos": demon of sleep.

Incidently, before he performed surgery, he made use of it to operate on the sick without pain (anesthesia did not exist at that time).

AUGUSTE AMBROISE LIÉBEAULT

A country doctor and co-founder of the Nancy School, he discovered the therapeutic value of hypnosis. He made use of it in consultation. He told his clients:

"Medicine is expensive. Hypnotherapy is free".

A persuasive argument, to which most submitted with goodwill.

Here is the way to apply his method:

The patient, installed in a comfortable armchair, directs his gaze towards yours. Reassure him that you know your subject. Give him confidence, and then command:

"Clear your head of everything. Don't think of anything anymore".

His attention is concentrated entirely on observing you. The other senses melt away, little by little becoming unable to capture external impressions.

Then speak to him of the different levels preceding sleep: fatigue, heaviness of the body, especially the eyelids, like this:

"Now your eyelids are getting heavy . . . Soon, they will close . . . Your vision is becoming blurred . . . Your arms and legs are getting heavier and heavier . . . Your body is heavy . . . My voice is going farther away . . . You are more and more tired . . . Now, your eyes have difficulty in staying open".

The patient closes his eyes. In the event of failure, repeat the suggestions and gently close his eyes.

Command:

"You are in a deep sleep!"

The word "sleep" brings about the hypnotic state after two minutes have elapsed. Begin the suggestive therapy.

Note: naive people, soldiers and children used to obedience are much more easily influenced.

Often, the simple command, "Sleep", will suffice.

H. BERNHEIM

Bernheim became interested in Liébeault's work and studied the phenomenon of hypnosis. He instituted hypnotherapy at the Nancy clinic. This was the beginning of the scientific application of hypnosis.

Dr. Cannon presents the application of Bernheim's methodology in the following order:

1. I sit the patient down in a comfortable armchair.

2. I command him to look into my eyes for the duration of one minute.

3. I tell him in a gentle, monotone (but firm) voice:

   a) everything will go very well

   b) your eyes are watering

c) your eyelids are becoming heavy

*d) a beneficial warmth envelops your
    arms and legs*

4. I command the patient to concentrate on the index finger and thumb of my left hand; I lower my hand at the same time (his eyelids will follow the movement).

5. If his eyes close, I have succeeded in the experiment.

6. If they do not close, I command:

"Close your eyes!"

7. I lift one of the patient's arms. I press it against the wall or against his head. I say,

"Your arm is stiff . . . Your head attracts it like a magnet".

8. If the effect is delayed, I repeat the suggestions.

9. My suggestion becomes more precise and more intense.

10. I suggest the absolute emptiness of thought, the conditioning of nervous reflexes and a feeling of well-being, rest and drowsiness.

11. As soon as one or another of these suggestions begins to take effect, I repeat it. I make sure

that the patient really feels the suggested sensations. Question him. If he nods his head, he means yes. If he shakes his head, he means no.

12. Each positive suggestion is important. Say:

"You are feeling quite well . . . Your arm is stiffening more and more. Now you can no longer lower it".

13. If the patient still moves his arm, I repeat:

"If you try to lower your arm, it will be blocked at the level of your head . . . Feel it. I am pulling your arm towards your head".

14. If the arm still does not stiffen, (which tells me that I have a too-skeptical patient), I halt the experiment.

15. The patient should never concentrate for too long on an object. One minute at the most.

16. Sometimes, it is enough to look at the patient for a second or two. At the same time, I offer my suggestions. Sleep follows. If not, I add:

"Sleep now!"

I pass my hand over his eyes. The hypnosis is a success.

The merit of Professor Bernheim lies in having given a precise definition of hypnosis; and in having instituted hypnosis by the spoken word, which is the basis of modern hypnosis.

J.M. CHARCOT

Charcot was chief physician at La Salpétrière, a professor of pathological anatomy and a neurologist with a world-wide reputation.

Charcot opposed the Nancy School and refuted its theories. According to him, hypnosis is not accomplished by the hypnotist. His definition: hypnosis is equivalent to an hysteric reaction.

His procedure was to induce strong reactions by spectacular means: by causing the sudden flashing of a cold light, causing a firecracker to explode, or by breaking silence with the unexpected ringing of a gong.

The sick and startled patients he treated fell under hypnosis in groups.

But since he treated only the mentally ill, he formulated a false opinion of hypnosis. In spite of his erroneous ideas, however, he occupies an important place as a seeker in this field.

His motto, "Only faith cures", is still true.

Charcot's method can be defined as "Hypnosis on signal". It precedes by more than half a century the "conditioned reflex" of Pavlov.

E. KRETSCHMER

Professor Ernst Kretschmer attempted to classify, in a scientific manner, the factors likely to induce hypnosis.

1. Relaxation:

    The patient detaches himself from everything except the object of concentration.

2. Ocular concentration:

    The patient, insensitive to all external stimuli, concentrates on an object placed near his eyes.

3. Conditioning:

    The hypnotist proceeds by repetition. Very precise suggestions are formulated and repeated exactly the same way each time. This method allows the therapist to make the patient always react in the same manner each time he repeats these suggestions. In this way, the hypnotist eliminates all feelings of insecurity.

4. Hypnosis: final goal.

The hypnotist now deepens the sleep state called hypnosis. The suggestions take root in the patient's subconscious. Further accomplishment: this brings out, in image form, events hidden at the bottom of the patient's memory. Pictured reminiscences of childhood are linked to your goal. The active cooperation of the patient is, of course, indispensable.

5. Help:

Any change — even for the better — causes apprehension in the patient. Therefore, give him a "help" signal — such as raising a finger — that you can respond immediately to with a brief command that all is well. Kretchmer believes that such reassuring peremptory commands are instinctively carried out by the subconscious, stimulated in this case by the logic of the conscious mind.

The hypnotic process of Kretschmer engages the patient in a close and active cooperation with the therapist. This is the current notion of the doctor-patient relationship.

EMILE COUÉ

Coué knew Liébeault in Nancy in 1885. He studied his theories on hypnosis. The Coué method is basically autosuggestion. It says that every hypnosis is really self-hypnosis (autosuggestion).

According to Coué, the hypnotist creates an idea in the patient's mind. This image then takes root in the subconscious. The subconscious, being a docile worker, transforms it into a spontaneous autosuggestion. Thus the idea becomes reality.

Every afternoon, people of every description met in his small conference room. The sessions were free. First he said a friendly word to each person there, and then Coué made this speech:

"Ladies and gentlemen, I am neither a doctor nor a health practitioner and I am certainly not a magician.

"I am going to explain to you my doctrine of autosuggestion and its practical application. But my method does not preclude medical treatment. I do not wish to, nor can I, replace the physician. I would like to place in your hands, and in theirs, an important remedy.

"Let us leave medical knowledge aside. I would like to teach you the following things — how to counteract humors and impulses; how to become a master in the

education of yourselves and your children.

"Do not underestimate the power of imagination. The insomniac imagines he cannot sleep; he would like to, but his imagination prevents him. The stammerer would like to be able to speak fluently; the asthmatic would like to breathe freely even in dense fog. There also, the imagination is dominant. The will says, 'I want to.' The imagination replies, 'I cannot'".

THE POWER OF THE IMAGINATION

Coué's theory.

"I'm going to present to you the risks you run if you let your imagination rule you. Perform this experiment. Make a fist. Close it very tightly, so tightly that you begin to shake. Think, 'I want to open this fist, but I can't do it, I can't do it.'

"Make the effort, all the while thinking, 'I can't do it'. You will not succeed. Now

say, 'I can do it'. You will finally open your fist."

Coué executed passes over painful and unhealthy parts of patients' bodies. At the same time, he said:

"The illness has disappeared". (Or, "it's going away".)

In fact, the pain ceased or at least the patient felt relief. The majority came away cured.

METHOD FOR INDUCING DEEP HYPNOSIS

Coué was essentially concerned with his doctrine of autosuggestion. But his method of inducing deep hypnosis should also be retained. It is described in his book, *"Hypnotic Sleep and Its Relation to Suggestion".*

How is it done?

Make a shiny object swing from right to left. Command the patient to follow the movement with his eyes, but without moving his head. Suggest:

"Think very hard, 'I want to sleep'... Feel it. You are falling asleep while following the movement of the object ... Your arms, your legs, your whole body grows heavy ... Your eyelids are heavy ... Heavier and heavier ... As

*heavy as lead ... Everything around
you grows dark ... Your eyes are watering ... You can see nothing but the object ... Sleep is overcoming you ... Now,
I will count up to twenty ... As I count,
your need for sleep will grow greater ...
Your eyes will be closed before the number twenty ... You are in a deep sleep".*

If on the number twenty the patient is not asleep,
command:

"Close your eyes! Sleep!"

Add deepening suggestions:

*"Now sleep ... You are in a deep
sleep ... Your sleep is deeper and
deeper ... Deeper and deeper".*

O. WETTERSTRAND

Wetterstrand, a Stockholm physician, and a pupil of
the Nancy School, stated that a person will involuntarily
adopt the "tics" of another if he observes them closely.
From this fact, he developed his principle, "mental contagion", which, according to him, is the basis of hypnotherapy.

He also inaugurated group hypnosis.

Every afternoon, Dr. Wetterstrand received forty people. They were distributed among three separate rooms, furnished at random with a large number of couches, armchairs and comfortable seats.

His procedure was to make use of the fascination method and begin with patients already successfully hypnotized in a previous session.

Even the most skeptical are apt to succumb to the effect of this method. This is applied to them in the presence of hypnotized subjects: mental contagion.

Wetterstrand went from one person to another. He would suggest to this one, "Your stomach pains are disappearing", to that one, "You no longer suffer from insomnia", etc. He reassured, relaxed them.

He applied the same method to all his patients who attained varying intensities of hypnosis, from deep hypnosis to simple relaxation. Wetterstrand deduced from this that the degree of depth of hypnosis had no effect on patients' reactions. Often the suggestions were carried out even at the level of simple relaxation.

Another of his opinions: hypnosis alone, by itself, is not enough to effect a cure. Such a cure would also depend on the receptivity of the patient to healing suggestions.

Wetterstrand triggered deep hypnosis by means of drugs, barbiturates, etc. In a house specially designed for it, he cared for drug addicts and alcoholics. They remained for days, even weeks at a time under hypnosis. Without coming out of hypnotic sleep for even a moment, they submitted to daily hypnotherapy.

GROSSMAN

His method, using effective little "tricks", is applied in the following manner:

First, I condition the receptivity of the patient. Half seated, half prone, he observes me. For several seconds. I suggest to him a feeling of warmth in his body, and heaviness in his arms resting on his knees.

At the same time, I seize his wrists, raise them slightly, then let them fall, telling him that they are as heavy as lead. Great fatigue slowly overcomes the patient. If his eyes do not yet reveal the fixedness required for the command: "Sleep!" I use the following trick:

I command the patient to close his eyes, or I close them for him. His arms are stretched upwards at right angles. I grasp his wrists. I suggest immense fatigue. Little by little, unable to hold himself in the seated position, he begins to sway backward. I encourage this movement by exerting slight pressure on his wrists. Throughout this procedure, the patient's head should rest on the armrest of the couch.

If necessary, I then command:

"Sleep".

All of the patients experience an irresistible fatigue. I explain, for example:

"Let yourself fall backwards from the sitting to the lying position. You will feel a slight dizziness, and a feeling of fatigue".

This experiment should last no longer than ten to twenty seconds.

Another "trick" is the Wetterstrand procedure:

With the patient settled comfortably, have him close his eyes. Pass your hand several times over his forehead, then descend to the pit of his stomach and exert light pressure.

Slow the rhythm of the pressures as you descend.

THE "RIFFAT" PROCEDURE

This is a medical experiment.

Hold a mask soaked with chloroform or chlorethylene in front of the patient's face. Result: a light narcosis.

If necessary, add one or two more drops. At the same time, make the appropriate suggestions.

Another way to do it is to simply put your hand under the patient's nose. Describe the smell of one or another of the products mentioned above. Accompany the gesture with adequate suggestions, like this:

"The smell is becoming stronger and stronger . . . Stronger and stronger".

The patient collapses.

If you have to deal with skeptics, give them the command to sleep. Pass your hand over their eyes. Variation: repeat the suggestions of heaviness; exert light pressures on the part of the body in question.

A. BRAUCHLE

Alfred Brauchle was chief physician of several large hospitals in succession. He had a thousand sessions to his credit and up to five hundred people might attend one of them. His scientific observations are recorded in numerous works.

In his book: *Hypnosis and Autosuggestion,* (Stuttgart 1961), he states:

"To my knowledge, no psychotherapy can be of help to so many patients at once. These sessions at which five hundred are present are meant to treat the subject. But, above all, each of them must find there his psychic 'help' and learn to apply it to himself as a miracle remedy. The close relationship between physiotherapy and psycho-therapy brings about a satisfactory result".

Note: All those present had been examined and treated physically before undergoing hypnotherapy.

Here is a typical experiment:

A patient, 21 years of age, paralyzed for two years, could neither sit down nor move his head. Cause: a possible cerebral tumor. An hypnosis is performed: no tumor.

I conclude from this that many physical illnesses are the effect of a psychic cause or conflict. The mind creates and cures illnesses. Materialism, wholly accepted just a few years ago, appears to be greatly compromised. We have lived and suffered too much not to believe in the powers of the mind.

INDIAN HYPNOSIS

THE INDIAN ROPE TRICK

Travellers relate the "supernatural" powers of Indian Yogis. And who has not heard of the symbolic snake-charmer, of the famous Indian rope trick?

Here is a description of this rope trick. The spectators gather around a fakir seated on the ground. A child of about twelve is seated next to him. His master seizes a coiled rope, throws it into the air. It remains fixed there.

The boy climbs it, and disappears from the spectators' view.

The fakir calls the child, urges him to return. No reply. Then there is a new command, and again the boy does not reply. Annoyed, a knife between his teeth, the master goes up the rope and . . . also disappears.

Suddenly, there a macabre shout. A moment later, the child's head falls to the ground. His arms, legs and torso follow. The fakir, covered with blood, slides down the rope. He picks up the scattered parts of the boy, puts them in a bag, and leaves.

He takes a few steps . . . the interior of the sack begins to move. The fakir puts down his load, opens it. The child stands up unharmed and runs away.

MASS SUGGESTION

Photograph these events. Surprise! The fakir and the child remain on the ground. The rope is thrown lengthwise along the ground; the urchin swarms along it on all-fours.

Why do these fearful phenomena seem to take place? Because the suggestive power of the fakir gives concrete form to the mental images of these events suggested to the subconscious minds of the spectators.

It is the transfer of one imagination to another, a power that is latent in every individual.

HOW CAN YOU DRAW ON THE POWER OF IMAGINATION?

First learn to give a form to your ideas. Here is a very simple exercise. Make a mental image of some object. Observe an object — say, a particular vase or a particular chair — placed before you. Command your "psychic eye" to make an image of it.

Carry out the following control:

Open your eyes, observe the object, close your eyes. Compare the concrete object with your mental image. Continue opening and closing your eyes until the object is reproduced in every detail and in every color.

If it is possible for you — after this training — to retain a mental image for a long time, and to retain it distinctly, you can attempt to transfer it to the imagination of someone else. Here is how:

Place such a person in front of you. Urge him to think of nothing in particular. Concentrate rigidly on some object that you have already engraved into your imagination.

HOW CAN THE TRANSFER OF IMAGINATION BE ACCOMPLISHED?

Close your eyes. "Will" the person to perceive your mental image of the object chosen. Your thought must impose it on his mind. Then ask the patient for a description of the object.

Note: He must be passive. If he tries to "will" the image to come to him, instead of calmly waiting for it to emerge in his mind, he will block it. In other words, any effort on his part leads to failure.

Important: keep nothing in your mind except the image. See it again and again and again as you are sending it to him.

The patient must be able to calm himself to receive it. Therefore, first check his eyes to measure this calm. Their lids should be slightly heavy. If not, relax him with the suggestions given earlier.

Once you start to gain control over the method, you can accomplish the transfer of more and more complex images. Persevere until you succeed with particularly skeptical people.

Remember that your training in mentally transferring images will continue over the years. Do not despair if your first attempts fail. One becomes a "fakir" only after many years of training.

Slowly widen your field of transfer to allow you to subjugate a group of people, and to impose a series of mental images, (events that unfold like a movie).

A STARTLING EVENT

A very skeptical European and an Indian healer were conversing on the shores of a lake infested with croaking frogs, concerning the reality of hypnotic powers. Tired of the discussion, the healer commanded the frogs to be quiet. And . . . they became quiet!

He added:

"They will be silent until tomorrow morning".

And the European only heard them resume their croaking the following morning.

THE POSTHYPNOTIC COMMAND

Intrigued, the European then asked the healer to re-peat the experiment the following evening. When the new command was given, there was a new silence!

A battery-powered recorder hidden on the shore had recorded the incantation and, of course, the continued croaking of the frogs! We conclude from this that the Eu-ropean — now deaf to the croaking — was under the posthypnotic influence of the command given.

But don't believe that these gifts are the exclusive province of the Indians! Try, persevere. You will do as much!

I happened to put a very skeptical person into deep hypnosis . . . after 28 sessions! Patience and perseverance overcome the worst obstacles.

If I tell you, "Every individual is hypnotizable", I am naturally thinking of normal people.

INDIAN METHOD USED
TO INDUCE HYPNOSIS

Here is a very effective Indian method which, unfortunately, is also very tiring for the hypnotist.

Required positions: the patient is lying on a reclining chair (the head portion slightly inclined). The face of the hypnotist is held directly above that of the subject. (Use of the fascination method.)

It is necessary to observe absolute silence and to detach oneself from the surroundings.

Here is how it's done: lower your head towards that of the patient. Stop at a distance of four to five inches. Maintain this position for from one to two hours. Think strongly, "The patient is falling asleep, he is concentrating on this idea".

To achieve an effect, wait thirty minutes, at the end of which the person's eyelids will start blinking. I advise you not to issue a counter-command. Command by thought only. If your concentration is not strong enough, strengthen the thought commands by appropriate suggestions.

This method, while infallible, requires an enormous power of concentration. The effort may have to be sustained for hours.

Therefore, I mainly include it here for your information. The other methods given you will almost invariable produce the same results.

THE FINGER PRESSURE METHOD

Here is another Indian method, effective and less demanding:

The patient is seated before you. You place your hands on his bare shoulders, one index finger on each side of the neck. Your thumbs meet at the nape of his neck.

Give the command to breathe slowly, regularly. Imperceptibly increase the pressure of your fingers. Wait a few minutes, the patient will manifest a need to sleep. Withdraw your fingers from his neck. Deepen the hypnosis thus triggered by appropriate suggestions. Determine the propitious moment for your commands by observing the relaxation of his neck muscles.

This method has proved effective where others have failed.

MORE DETAILS ABOUT YOUR PRACTICE IN THE HYPNOSIS OF SELF AND OTHERS

RAPPORT

I have developed this theme and its procedure in the chapter, "How do you initiate a consultation?" I will describe it to you here in greater detail.

By "rapport", I mean the contact established between you and your patient. He must be detached from his surroundings, so he can concentrate exclusively on your voice.

Often you can create the so-called "isolated rapport". In this case, he is subject only to your influence. He remains deaf to any suggestions formulated by a third party.

How is this isolated rapport produced? Either spontaneously under hypnosis, or by appropriate suggestions.

CAN THE RAPPORT BE BROKEN?

I reply: yes. The rapport can be broken — which means a loss of contact between him and you.

Under what circumstances? If you are dealing with a psychically passive individual, he may increase the depth of your hypnosis by autosuggestion, until he sinks into himself alone. . . isolated within himself alone.

Another negative outcome: you may be confronted by an truly introverted human being, incapable of concentrating on your voice.

These cases are rare and should not cause you to lose your wits. For example, you notice that the patient under hypnosis has slipped out of your control. He no longer reacts to your suggestions.

Keep your cool. Above all, do not break off the hypnosis. This would be a fundamental error. Deepen the hypnosis instead, with the help of adequate suggestions.

How do you re-establish contact?

Make circular passes over his forehead and his whole body. Say:

"You are quite calm . . . Your breathing is slow, regular . . . You are sinking deeply into a state of peace and relaxation . . . Feel it. You feel quite well . . . One moment, you have turned your attention towards yourself . . . Now you hear me distinctly . . . Concentrate on my voice . . . Your hypnotic state is almost

over ... We will break it off together. Do not let yourself be distracted ... Concentrate on my voice ... Nothing else is important ... Feel it. A wonderful freshness envelops your body ... Your arms, your legs are relaxed ... You are full of strength and energy ... In great shape ... Soon, I will count to three. On three, you will open your eyes ... You will feel fresh and alert ... One ... Two ... Three ... Open your eyes! Stretch out your arm. You are completely awake ... In top form".

Throughout my career, I have only encountered two ruptures of rapport.

To re-establish contact, I have proceeded as described above. Note that it is important to deepen the hypnosis before progressively lifting it.

HOW DO YOU GIVE ANOTHER PERSON CONTROL OVER THE PATIENT'S HYPNOSIS?

Put the patient under hypnosis by the usual means. Then make the following suggestions:

"From this moment, you will obey the commands of Mr. X as if they were mine. You will carry them out immediately. You cannot, nor do you want to act in any other way. This is rooted in your subconscious. You will obey Mr. X".

This suggestion conditions obedience even in the waking state. All commands given by Mr. X to the patient outside the hypnotic state will be instantly carried out.

Here is some final advice: when you are transferring hypnotic control, avoid any word or gesture which would later accidentally set off hypnosis. The suggestions of Mr. X should never have the effect of posthypnotic commands.

Naturally, this control may also be transferred to a woman.

HOW TO PRACTICE SELF-HYPNOSIS BY EXCHANGE OF CONTROL

As you can see, any compotent hypnotist can transfer control to you. In this way, he gives you posthypnotic commands, which you can then use to hypnotize yourself.

This is especially fruitful when you have any difficulty in hypnotizing yourself. Here's how it is done:

The hypnotist begins by putting you under hypnosis. Then he transfers the rapport — the control — to you, while giving you a code word. After this, whenever you speak this word, you will automatically fall into a hypnotic state.

This indirect procedure provides an excellent gateway into your first self-hypnosis.

ADAPTATION TO THE PATIENT

HOW DO YOU DEVELOP STANDARD TECHNIQUES?

Your experiments are to be carried out by means of the different techniques proposed in this method. Some of them will suit you perfectly. Others will not work. Select the best from each of them and make a synthesis. This will be your standard method to trigger hypnosis — your personal, infallible method.

Nevertheless, you may at any time meet a patient who will react less well to your method. What do you do in this case? Adapt it to his motivations.

HOW DO YOU ADAPT YOUR METHOD TO THE PATIENT?

The first question to put to him is the following:

"Have you been hypnotized? By which method?"

If he has, an imprint and a certain tolerance will remain with him from it. He therefore may not yield to your method, considering it to be unthinkable and erroneous.

Your method — until you correct it — will be ineffective.

There are two other important factors to consider. His state of mind, and the motivation that led him to consult you.

Let's begin with his state of mind. He may confuse the hypnotic state with unconsciousness. Therefore, when he is put under hypnosis, he will feel taken advantage of. It has not corresponded to his expectations. The depth of the hypnosis will therefore be shallow.

His conduct is motivated by certain hopes, It is up to you to discover them and to adapt to them as best you can.

ADAPTING TO THE LANGUAGE AND INTELLECTUAL LEVEL OF THE PATIENT

It is very important to formulate suggestions according to his language and intellectual level. These suggestions will be effective only if he understands them, and if they respond to the language of his subconscious (and can therefore be transformed into mental images in his mind).

Therefore, different methods will suit different patients. As a consequence, hypnosis must be adapted to each individual.

What qualities must you have to do this?

A great deal of tact and sensitivity. Plus the patience and ability to identify with his personality. Without this making of his personality your own, your influence will be seriously compromised.

I will show you how to do this below.

HOW DO YOU PROJECT YOUR PERSONALITY INTO HIS?

It is also important to hypnotically project your personality, through hypnosis, into his mind. Those characteristics you wish can then be transferred to him.

Let his welfare dominate this exchange. Do not seek your own ends. If this condition is respected, you will automatically create a trusting atmosphere. The patient will allow himself to be manipulated without prejudice.

The experience necessary to be able to guess, in a few minutes of observation, the personality and problems of the patient, is acquired. Practice of the techniques below will allow you to form, in a few seconds, an idea of his situation, his hopes, his concerns.

THE PATIENT DESCRIBES HIS WISHES

During the first session, the patient will make known his confused and ill assorted wishes. You must then organize this information into a comprehensive and intelligible image, that is easily rooted in the subconscious.

How do you sort out your suggestions? Let me quote you an example.

Let us suppose that the patient describes his desires as follows:

"Above all, I would like to be rid of my headaches, of my insomnia. For years I have had to use sedatives. I wake up every night. I can't get back to sleep.

"In the daytime, I am in the grip of anxieties and I get very tired. Sometimes my heart beats so fast, it feels as if it wants to jump out of my chest. I have lost all confidence in myself. I am subject to depressions which last for days. I can't look people in the eye anymore. I can't bear them in a restricted space like an elevator. I run away!"

HOW DO YOU TRANSFORM THIS INFORMATION INTO SUGGESTIONS?

Let us begin by transforming simple information into effective suggestions.

Here are some examples.

Information: "Above all I would like to be rid of my headaches . . ."

Suggestion:

"Your head is clear, freed of all pain".

Information: " . . . to be rid of my insomnia . . . "

Suggestion:

"Every evening, as soon as you are in bed, all worrisome thoughts will leave you. A feeling of peace and harmony will envelop you. You will instantly fall asleep. Your sleep will be sound, natural, wholesome. You will sleep deeply every night. Upon waking, you will still experience this feeling of peace and harmony. You will be happy and content".

Information: "In the daytime, I am in the grip of anxieties and I get very tired . . . "

Suggestion:

"You are quite calm . . . Quite calm . . . You are feeling quite well".

Information: "Sometimes, my heart beats so fast, it feels as if it wants to jump out of my chest . . . "

Suggestion:

"Your heart is beating slowly, regularly. Its rhythm is calm, regular. Your circulation is excellent. Feel your well-being in every situation".

Information: "I have lost all confidence in myself. I am subject to depressions which last for days".

Suggestion:

"Your assurance and your confidence in yourself grow day by day. Feel it. You are more and more sure of yourself. You have more and more confidence in yourself. You feel quite at ease in any situation".

Information: "I can't look people in the eye anymore".

Suggestion:

"You like to mix with people. You seek out their company. You look everyone straight in the eye".

Information: "I can't bear them in a restricted space like an elevator. I run away".

Suggestion:

"You seek out the company of others. You feel at ease in a group of people. Nothing can convince you to the contrary".

HOW YOU DEVELOP
A GLOBAL SUGGESTION

You can bring together all the suggestions given into a global suggestion. For example:

"You are quite calm ... A wonderful feeling of peace and harmony spreads through your body ... Feel it. You are happy and content. Your assurance and confidence in yourself grow day by day ... Day by day, you are more and more sure of yourself ... Feel your well-being in your situation ... Your heart beats slowly, regularly ... Your circulation is excellent ... You seek out the company of others ... You look everyone straight in the eye ... In the midst of a group of people, you feel at ease ... Free of all complexes ... Your head is clear ... Your heart beats calmly ... Your assurance and self-confidence grow day by day .... Nothing can make you ill-at-ease any longer".

FORMULATIONS WHICH FLOW FROM THE PRECEDING ONES

I have just brought various suggestions together into a single global suggestion. I recommend that you do this as a matter of course. That you take all the information each patient gives you, and you build them together into one global suggestion.

When you have finished with this overall string of images, take a moment of silence to recover your creative faculties.

However, do not allow this prolonged pause to occur without giving a suggestion that tells the patient what to do while it is happening. Otherwise, the rapport — shall we say the spell — will be broken.

Here are some examples of suggestions before a pause:

"You are breathing calmly, freely".

"You are breathing slowly, regularly ... You are feeling quite well".

"Nothing distracts you ... You are to wait ... Wait for my voice to return once more".

"You have no more desires ... You are quite passive ... Let yourself be carried

along ... Let yourself go ... Nothing is important".

"Feel it. You are quite well ... You are sinking more and more into this feeling of peace and well-being".

If these suggestions are given in this sequence, you may allow yourself a pause, to deepen the hypnosis.

HOW DO YOU MANUFACTURE AND THEN OVERCOME A TERRIFYING FICTITIOUS EVENT?

Here is another interesting technique. You confront the patient under hypnosis with a situation he is terrified of in everyday life.

Let us use the example of a patient who is afraid of people in general, and especially afraid of them in an elevator.

This information allows you to formulate the following suggestion:

"You feel quite calm, free ... You are feeling quite well ... You are in the center of a huge hotel lobby. Around you are small groups of people. Some are engaged in discussion. Others are moving

in this direction or that. There is an elevator not very far from you. Its door opens. You see your friend there. You go to join him. He says that he is going to the restaurant on the top floor. You go with him. You rejoice at this fortunate chance meeting.

"At each floor, people leave the elevator. Others enter. This movement makes no difference to you. You are happy to have the opportunity of spending a pleasant moment with your friend. In the restaurant there is a free place. You take it. It's a sunny day. A magnificent panorama is spread out at your feet.

"You order your snack. You remember that you were calm, free of any complexes in the elevator. You felt at ease there. It made no difference to you to be among so many people. You are proud of yourself, relieved. Your friend has to leave. You pay the bill. You go back down in the elevator.

"One floor down, a group of tourists enters the elevator. You are all crowded

together. Their gaiety is contagious. Having arrived at the destination, everyone rushes out. Such shoving! But you remain serene, at ease. You say goodbye to your friend, then leave.

"Now, taking the elevator seems to be the most natural thing in the world. In future, it will all happen in reality as you have JUST lived it in your imagination".

HOW DO YOU TRANSFORM FICTION INTO REALITY?

If this suggestion is repeated as often as necessary — especially if it is recorded on a tape — the event will become part of the patient's personality. It will become automatic. It will be registered by the subconscious which will no longer make the distinction between fiction and reality. The patient will adopt the desired conduct.

It is important to separate the overall problem into several successive stages. In this case, first the fear of the elevator was dealt with . . . then the fear of people . . . then going up in the elevator . . . then going down . . . then being jostled . . . etc. All the patient's fears and/or desires are to be treated separately.

IN WHAT TONE OF VOICE MUST SUGGESTIONS BE MADE?

If you give, for example, a suggestion of peace in an irritated, hurried voice, you will obtain no result. But if you say it in a calm, monotonous voice, and lower your tone at the end of the sentence, the patient will immediately relax.

Your voice must be neither too strong nor too muted. Your tone must be neither raucous nor shrill. It must betray no hesitation — which might seriously compromise the required impression of absolute assurance.

Work to maintain mastery over your whole person. This is the decisive factor. Through this, you will lead the patient to believe in your gifts.

METHODS EFFECTIVE FOR DEEPENING HYPNOSIS

The simplest, most effective method for deepening hypnosis is to observe a few minutes of silence.

The patient must not fall asleep during this time. Here is a suggestion for keeping the patient awake:

"I will soon be silent. During this silence, you will breathe slowly, regularly. With each breath, you will sink more

deeply under hypnosis. At the end of five minutes, it will be deeper than before. If I start speaking again, you will hear me distinctly. You will obey me".

After five minutes have gone by, the patient will be under deep hypnosis. He will hear you clearly. Continue the hypnosis.

Here is a very effective variation: hypnosis under hypnosis.

Put a patient under hypnosis. When he starts to pass control to you, tell him to imagine himself being put under hypnosis again.

When his hypnosis deepens, tell him to imagine that he is being put under hypnosis still again.

You thus have the means to make him undergo several successive hypnoses.

EXAMPLES OF SEVERAL SUCCESSFUL HYPNOSES UNDER HYPNOSIS

FIRST PHASE

Trigger the hypnosis by means of the usual procedures. Suggest:

"Now, your psychic eye is going to make a mental image of everything I will tell you. Picture it. You come to me for consultation. I receive you at the door. Together we enter the room set aside for the practice of hypnosis. I ask you to lie down comfortably. You picture yourself in that position. Your breathing is calm, regular... With each breath you sink into the pleasant feeling brought about by the hypnotic state. I leave you for a moment without speaking to you.

"Your hypnosis is deep. You feel as if you are sinking still more deeply into the hypnotic state. Picture it. Now, I come toward you. I give you the desired suggestions. You are receptive to my words. Feel it. They are taking root in your personality. You will carry them out to the letter. Listen to me. I will now slowly raise your hypnosis. I will count to three. On three, you will open your eyes. Your will stretch your arms. You will be in great form".

SECOND PHASE

*"I am going to put you into a second
hypnotic state. Feel it. I am passing my
hand over your forehead, over your
arms ... Your eyes, your arms are becoming as heavy as lead. You are
breathing calmly, regularly. At each
breath, you are sinking more and more
into this wonderful feeling of fatigue
and heaviness.*

*"Feel it. This fatigue is overcoming you.
You feel safe. This hypnosis is deeper
than those that preceded it. My voice
comes to you from far off, but you hear it
distinctly. Nothing is more important ...
You want to rest ... You surrender to
this pleasant feeling of heaviness and fatigue. Absorbed in this wonderful, peaceful state, you listen to me as I give you
the desired suggestions. My words are
branded into your memory and your
subconscious. You are convinced that
you cannot forget them.*

*"I leave you for a moment in this hyp-
notic state without speaking to you. Dur-*

ing this time, my words take still deeper root in your subconscious. You will carry out my commands.

"Your psychic eye sees you lying down in this condition. Feel it. This hypnosis is deeper than any other. You can see how I come towards you. Listen to me. I am progressively lifting the hypnosis. You have the feeling of returning from another world. A well-being that is beyond words has taken possession of you."

(The patient now seems capable of undergoing a third, even-deeper hypnosis under hypnosis).

HOW DO YOU RAISE THE HYPNOSIS?

The patient is still under deep hypnosis. But now, it must be finished. Give him these suggestions:

"Soon, I will count to three. On three, your arms and legs will be flexible. You will open your eyes. You will feel fresh and alert. One ... Two ... Three ... Open your eyes.

"Feel it. You are fresh and alert. Your arms and legs are flexible once more.

Move them. Stretch them. Stand up. You are full of strength and energy".

HOW DO YOU LEAD HIM TO DEEPEN THE HYPNOSIS BY MAKING HIM SPEAK AND WRITE UNDER HYPNOSIS?

First suggest:

"Your hypnosis is deep, but you can talk".

Then the patient will repeat the important suggestions given under the hypnosis ten to twenty times.

Suggest that he open his eyes, without leaving the hypnotic state. Next, tell him:

"With each word you write, your hypnosis will grow deeper".

Here is another very effective procedure: self-hypnosis. If you yourself are under hypnosis, the effect of your suggestions will be strengthened. I personally make use of this method.

GOING BACKWARDS IN TIME

A most rewarding hypnotic phenomenon is transporting someone into the past. Suggest to him that he is of a certain age. Three years old, for instance. Put him under hypnosis. His behavior will be consistent with the mentality of that age. Better yet, he will remember all events, in the smallest detail.

Rare is the person capable — in the waking state —of describing in such detail the dress his mother was wearing on a given day. But under hypnosis, they will not only be able to do this, but will relate who came to visit shortly before noon.

The events of any given period return all together, accompanied by a host of details. All the senses are awake: smell, hearing, etc.

This corroborates the following fact: our subconscious records even the most insignificant details of past events. It stores and preserves them forever, even if our conscious mind no longer has the slightest memory of them.

TOTAL TRANSFERENCE THROUGH TIME

We identify two ways to go back in time. The first is total transference: the patient no longer has any memory whatever of his real age. If he is projected into earliest infancy, he will behave as he did then.

One day, I put a twenty-two year old journalist under hypnosis. I suggested to him:

"You are three years old. You will come with me to the basement".

Instinctively, he gave me his hand and followed me. He went down the stairs as a child of three would. He always put the same foot on each step and brought the other one behind it.

PARTIAL TRANSFERENCE

This second type of transference through time can be accomplished under light hypnosis. The patient relives the events of a suggested time in the past, all the while retaining the idea of the present time. We then have a kind of duality. Here are the elements of this:

1.The patient can speak to you. He is aware of your personality. He knows his real age.

2. But he simultaneously relives, in detail, the events of a past time; he provides precise information about it which will be used to discover the cause of an illness or disturbance.

A CASE STUDY

Four years ago, I cured a stutterer who had borne this cross since the age of eight.

Here is the reason. He took a trip with his parents. They had an auto accident. He was the only one unhurt. The guilt produced the stuttering.

At the time I undertook to treat him, he was twenty-four years old. I brought him progressively backwards in time. At each stage, he stuttered.

Finally, we arrived at his age at the time of the accident. And surprise! He no longer stuttered!

I then transferred the young man once more to his real age. He was cured!

How did I work this cure? I proceeded back to the time of the accident in small time steps. I took him back by progressive and repeated transfers.

By this method, he went back slowly to the accident several times. He finally — after approaching it slowly, and then living it over again and again — accepted it mentally.

In similar cases, I would advise you not to effect a total transference. Do not search directly for the time of trauma. The past event is still too vivid in his field of consciousness. You will cause a new trauma.

Instead, proceed by partial transference. Let him go back a few years at a time. This way, the patient, slowly approaching the time of the scene from the past, relives it as a spectator.

This method allows you to get rid of hidden, unassimilated traumas, with no risk of creating new inhibitions.

HOW DO YOU ACCOMPLISH A TRANSFERENCE TO ANOTHER LIFE?

Here is a curious variation of transference into the past. The patient returns slowly to his birth. Then, he is projected beyond in time.

For certain persons, I cause them to relive a former life. At least they described the existence of human beings who lived one, two or three hundred years ago. They all claimed, "We were this person".

No particular technique is required. It is enough to give appropriate suggestions and to progressively lead the patient through time.

TEST: HOW SENSITIVE WILL YOU — OR SOMEONE ELSE — BE TO HYPNOSIS?

According to one popular rule, every human being is suggestible, but not necessarily hypnosensitive. I do not agree.

With reference to my personal experience, I can state:

"Every sane individual can be hypnotized if he so wishes. It is simply necessary to bring about the required conditions."

DECISIVE FACTORS

Here is an essential condition: choose a time of day that corresponds to a fatigue phase. This will strengthen the suggestion of tiredness and heaviness.

Use the graph below to determine the propitious time. The curve represents the degrees of human activity, spread out over a normal day.

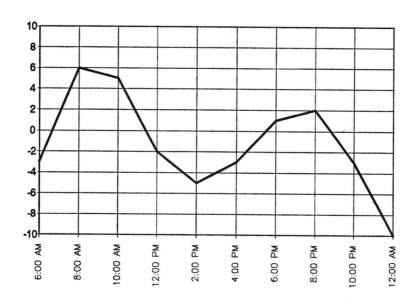

INSTRUCTIONS FOR THE TEST

To see how deeply your patients will go under hypnosis, do this:

Have them answer spontaneously with "yes" or "no" to the questions in the following test. Each "yes" scores one point. Are they unsure of a question? Put a "no". Add up their points.

Under six points: he is a difficult subject to hypnotize. But you can create favorable conditions which will allow him to be put under hypnosis. Your capacity for assimilation will allow you to gather enough information from him to formulate effective suggestions.

Does he have a total of more than five points? He will readily be hypnotized.

	TEST	*YES*	*NO*
1.	Do you practice relaxation exercises: Yoga, meditation, autogenic training?	☐	☐
2.	Are you able to relax at any time, even if you are tense?	☐	☐
3.	Do you make use of a routine to go to sleep?	☐	☐
4.	Do you sometimes live in an imaginary world which takes you far from reality?	☐	☐

		YES	*NO*
6.	Do you have an extravagant imagination?	☐	☐
7.	Do you have the ability to create mental images?	☐	☐
8.	Are you strongly impressed by pleasant events or images?	☐	☐
9.	When you follow a film, do you live the event intensely?	☐	☐
10.	Are your emotions spontaneous? Do they disappear as quickly as they came?	☐	☐
11.	If you have to wait, are you irritated, impatient?	☐	☐
12.	Do you let your impulses rule you?	☐	☐
13.	Do you let yourself be easily intimidated?	☐	☐
14.	According to you are you easily influenced?	☐	☐
15.	Do you allow yourself to be distracted when you work?	☐	☐
16.	Do you adopt a passive attitude when an important decision must be taken or responsibility assumed?	☐	☐
17.	Does the impressive appearance of your neighbor influence you?	☐	☐
18.	Do you like human contact?	☐	☐

<u>*YES*</u> <u>*NO*</u>

20. Do you have absolute confidence in cer- ☐ ☐
      tain people?

Now add up the "yes" answers. Score one point for each "yes".

From zero to four points: difficult to hypnotize.

From five to eleven points: moderately hypnosensitive.

From twelve to twenty points: very easy to hypnotize.

PERSONALITY MODIFICATIONS BY MEANS OF HYPNOSIS

MODIFICATIONS OF THE PERSONALITIES OF THE HYPNOTIST AND THE PATIENT

Hypnotizing a person for the first time is an unforgettable event. Success in transferring your will to an individual will endow you with an assurance that will be noticed by those around you. You will discover another dimension of your personality.

How can you succeed in this first effort? By choosing someone who is easy to hypnotize. Hypnosis offers you a whole gamut of procedures. You will develop your own personality while changing that of someone else.

But remember — if your goals are motivated by pride and selfishness, you will pay the price. His subconscious will be in opposition to your influence as an implacable judge.

TWO PERSONALITY MODIFICATIONS

First, there is the modification of our personality that takes place during our lifetime. Hypnotic transference back through time supplies us with proof of these types of changes — often, of course, unconscious.

Hypnosis gives you a very effective way of dealing with this modification. It can be brought about by returning the patient into his past, as shown above.

But it will also take place if we project the patient into the future. Transferred to the future, he will act according to the more socially and spiritually advanced age suggested. These fictitious degrees of maturity and personal development can be consolidated under hypnosis. The given behavior will definitely be acquired by the patient.

The second transformation of personality is immediate and takes place in the present.

I attended the transformation of personality of a student into a historic reality — Napoleon. Little by little, he adopted the physical manner, then the psychic manias of the emperor. Then, the psychologist suggested to him:

"Write the order of the day on a slate".

The student vehemently refused. The firm command of the psychologist countered this refusal. The patient wrote:

"Soldiers! If one has the audacity to command the emperor to write something on a slate, I resign! Napoleon".

This example shows to what extent we can identify with another's personality.

DELIBERATE CHANGE
IN CERTAIN QUALITIES

Under hypnosis, human qualities can be changed. Medical hypnosis has many proofs of this.

No particular technique is required. The hypnosis is triggered and the appropriate suggestions given. Let us suppose that you wish to project someone into the future to cure negative qualities. In this case, use the following suggestions.

HOW DO YOU PROJECT SOMEONE INTO
THE FUTURE?

"You are quite calm ... You are breathing slowly, regularly ... You are feeling quite well ... Your peace is profound ... Nothing distracts you ... Nothing is important anymore ... You listen only to my voice ... You will obey my commands ... You are twenty-five years old at the present time ... Feel it. You are growing older ... 26 ... 27 ... 28 ... 29 ... Now, you are thirty years old. Think, feel age thirty ... Your peace is profound ... You can speak to me ... You answer my questions ... You

remember in detail the events of the past five years."

These suggestions having been given, you can question the patient without prejudice to the degree of depth of the hypnosis.

But there is one condition required to obtain a success: deep hypnosis.

Not everyone is receptive to this type of hypnotic state. But throughout your career you will find patients who will be easily projected into the future.

AUTOMATIC WRITING

Take a pencil. Place the point lightly on a white sheet of paper. Your subconscious will tend to control the muscles of your hand. You will begin to write automatically. It will be possible for you to simultaneously read and carry on a conversation.

REQUIRED PREPARATIONS

Certain human beings who practice writing can write simultaneously with the left and right hands, all while they are holding a conversation. 15% to 20% are capable of performing this type of writing in the waking state. Under hypnosis, the percentage climbs to 80%.

Have you mastered self-hypnosis? If so, put yourself into a hypnotic state. If not, have yourself hypnotized. Sit down in a comfortable seat. Place a rigid cardboard on your knees. Put a sheet of paper on it, to which you softly hold the point of a pencil.

Order your subconscious to control your hand, to write on some given subject. (If you have been put under hypnosis, the hypnotist will give you the necessary suggestions.)

Trace broad circles on the paper for a minute. Always keep to the same rhythm. Then push your hand towards the edge of the sheet. Write:

"Now, I am beginning to write automatically. My hand writes without my intervention".

UNKNOWN HANDWRITING COMING FROM AN "ALIEN POWER"

Now ignore your hand. Look in another direction. You hand will write in a handwriting that is unknown to you.

If you do not immediately succeed, begin the exercise again. Little by little, your hand will become independent. A strange, disquieting sensation: an alien power seems to guide your hand!

On the first attempt, the sentences are close together, as though in a single word. Restart the experiment often, the automatic handwriting will become intelligible and readable.

MORE TESTS: HOW DO YOU CONTROL THE HYPNOSIS?

FIRST TEST: BLOCKAGE OF THE EYES

Once the hypnosis has been triggered, it is interesting to know to what extent the hypnotized person carries out your orders. To do this, you have several tests of your control at your disposal. These will be accompanied by appropriate suggestions.

Let us begin by having the patient close his eyes.

HOW DOES THE CLOSING OF THE EYES WORK?

Here is the suggestion:

"Feel it. Your eyelids are becoming heavy ... Heavier and heavier ... Your eyes are hermetically closed ... Now, you can no longer open them. You no longer want to ... Let yourself sink into this feeling of lassitude and heaviness that is overcoming you ... More and more ... You are very tired ... Your eyelids, as heavy as lead, seem to be glued ... You

can no longer open your eyes ... You no longer desire to do so ... Try it. You are incapable of it ... The more you struggle to open them, the more your eyes will close ... You are sinking more and more deeply into this feeling of lassitude and heaviness".

Do the person's eyes remain shut after this command has been twice repeated? If so, you may deduce that the hypnosis has taken effect. Observe the eye muscles and determine if the subject who has undergone the experiment is trying to open them.

HOW DO YOU APPLY THE TEST WITHOUT TRIGGERING HYPNOSIS?

Have you conditioned him to undergo hypnosis in the waking state? In this case, apply the test without triggering hypnosis, with the help of this suggestion:

"Now, please close your eyes. I will count to three. On three, you will try to open your eyes. You will be unable to do so. On three, you will no longer be able to open your eyes. One ... Two ... Three ... Feel it. You can no longer open your eyes ... Try ... The harder you try ...

*the less you will succeed ... Try
again ... You are incapable of it ...
Now, you can no longer open your eyes
at all".*

In spite of his efforts, the person should be unable to open his eyes. From that moment, it will be necessary to heighten the suggestion, like this:

*"I am counting to three ... On three you
will easily be able to open your eyes ...
One ... Two ... Three ... Open your
eyes! Feel it. Your eyelids feel light ...
Everything is normal again, as it was
before the test ... You can open your
eyes".*

It is indispensable to repeat each suggestion several times and to heighten each one separately.

SECOND TEST: BLOCKAGE OF THE ARMS

To perform this test, you suggest to the person:

"Your arms are heavy and immoveable".

Observe his reactions. You can judge by them the degree to which your suggestions have been recorded and carried out.

THE SUGGESTION

"You are surrendering to a pleasant feeling of lassitude and heaviness which overcomes you . . . Each one of your fingers is becoming as heavy as lead . . . Feel it. Your arms are heavy, immoveable . . . This heaviness overcomes your arms and your hands. You can no longer lift them . . . Feel it. Your arms are quite immoveable."

HOW DO YOU JUDGE?

Judge whether the person is trying to lift his arms. Observe the forearm muscles. They will relax. If the candidate can still lift his arms and hands, you may deduce that the hypnosis was effective but not deep enough. In this event, repeat the suggestion several times. You will, little by little, achieve the desired immobility.

Have you conditioned the person to undergo hypnosis in the waking state? The following suggestion will suffice to perform the test:

"I will soon count to three. On three, you will try to lift your arms. Once I have said the number three, you will not be able to make this movement. One . . .

Two ... Three ... Now, you can no longer lift your arms at all".

HOW DO YOU HEIGHTEN THIS SUGGESTION?

First, observe to what degree your suggestion has been carried out and whether the hypnosis has taken effect. Then, heighten it like this:

"I am counting to three once more. At three, you will be able to move your arms, Your arms will be flexible and mobile again ... Everything will be as it was before the test. You are feeling quite well. One ... Two ... Three ... Feel it. Your arms are flexible, light, mobile ... You are feeling quite well".

Question the candidate. Try to judge whether his arms are flexible. If not, the suggestion must be repeated.

THIRD TEST: THE FALL TO JUDGE HYPNOSENSITIVITY

Ask the person to place himself in the middle of the room.

With his eyes closed, he concentrates on his balance. Give the following suggestion:

"Keep your eyes closed ... Feel it. You feel flexible, light ... Try not to fall. Now, you are starting to fall backwards ... More and more ... The force that is pulling you grows stronger ... You can hardly resist it ... You are pulled backwards more and more".

How do you strengthen this effect? Place your right hand one inch behind the candidate's head, your left hand five inches in front of his eyes. Give the suggestion.

At the same time, perform the following movement: your right hand moves away from his head and your left is brought close to his face. Follow up with these suggestions:

"Feel it. You are falling. You no longer resist ... You are falling! ... Don't be afraid, I will catch you ... There is no danger ... You feel as though this force is pulling you irresistibly backward ... You are beginning to fall. Fall!"

People who are very suggestible will very quickly sway, then fall backwards.

HOW DO YOU APPLY THIS TEST UNDER HYPNOSIS IN THE POST-HYPNOTIC WAKING STATE?

Have you conditioned the candidate to undergo hypnosis in future waking states? Then the following suggestion will suffice to gain control:

> *"I will count to three . . . On three, you will feel yourself pulled backwards . . . You will not resist . . . On three, you will fall backwards . . . I will catch you . . . You will try to remain upright . . . The more you try, the more you will fall. One . . . Two . . . Three . . . You are beginning to fall backwards . . . Fall!"*

If the test has proven to be conclusive, heighten the suggestions given, as follows:

> *"I will soon count to three . . . On three, you will set yourself upright. No force will any longer be pulling you backwards. Everything will be normal again, as it was before the test. Your legs will hold you up solidly. One . . . Two . . . Three . . . See, you are upright!"*

FOURTH TEST: JOINING THE HANDS
HOW DO YOU JUDGE SUGGESTIBILITY?

This test, used by illusionists in large shows, allows very suggestible candidates to be selected.

They proceed in the following manner:

First, they ask the audience to cross the fingers of their two hands. Their hands are then placed in that position on top of their head. Then, they suggest:

"Your fingers are strongly entwined. I am soon going to count to three. On three, you will try to pull your fingers apart. You will not be able to do it. You will no longer be able to separate your hands. They will stick together. The more you try to separate them, the more they will be welded together. Now you can no longer separate them. One ... Two ... Three ... etc. ..."

This suggestion can be applied under hypnosis in the waking state. In this case, you will lift it as soon as the test is successful. Here are the appropriate phrases:

"I'm going to count to three ... On three you will separate your hands ... One ... Two ... Three ... Feel it. Your hands separate easily ... Everything is normal

again, as it was before the test ... Your hands are flexible and mobile".

HOW DO YOU COMBINE THIS TEST WITH A POSTHYPNOTIC COMMAND?

You can achieve the combination of test and posthypnotic command. This is applicable under hypnosis in the waking state, as follows:

"I am soon going to count to three. On three, you will cross the fingers of your two hands. You will no longer be able to separate them. One ... Two ... Three ... If you cross your fingers, you will no longer be able to separate them. Feel it. Your hands are welded together ... If I count to three again, you will be able to separate them. Your hands will be flexible and mobile once more. One ... Two ... Three ... Separate your hands. See, you can do it. Now, they are flexible and mobile".

FIFTH TEST: MEMORY INHIBITION

This test requires a hypnosis of medium depth. If you succeed in this, be assured that all your suggestions will be recorded and carried out.

As a security measure, you might put the person under deep hypnosis and give the following suggestion:

THE SUGGESTION

"From this moment on, your subconscious is registering all my words. You will obey me. Now, you will forget the number five. You can no longer remember it at all nor even say it. Surrender to this state of peace and relaxation which overcomes you. You are able to speak. If I command you to do so, you will count from one to ten, leaving out the number five. Count!"

If the candidate forgets the number five, you may heighten the suggestion by repeating it.

The test having been successful, heighten the suggestion as follows:

"The number five now returns to your memory. Everything is normal again, as

it was before the test. You remember the number five. You count from one to ten. You include the number five".

HOW DO YOU BLOCK OUT A WORD FROM MEMORY OR REPLACE IT BY ANOTHER?

Here is an amusing exercise. Replace, for instance, the number five by another word. This might be "zips". The candidate will count: one, two, three, four, zips, six, etc. Make him perform the following multiplication: "zips times zips make?"

You will get an answer like: "Twenty-zips".

Is the hypnosis deep? In this case, you can block out this word from memory or replace it by another. The person's name, for instance. This difficult exercise may cause tears and the gnashing of teeth. In this event, heighten the suggestion immediately.

Here is a variation: have you conditioned the candidate to submit to hypnosis in the waking state? Suggest to him that he no longer remembers his name. On three, he will struggle to think of it. Impossible! The spectators will claim it is a sham. However, the person will definitely no longer remember his name. Nevertheless, he will refuse to admit it.

SIXTH TEST: BLOCKAGE OF LANGUAGE

To perform this kind of test, a suggestion is made to the person that he can no longer say a certain word. His name, for example. The memory of this can become an obsession to the degree that he will be incapable of saying it.

THE SUGGESTION

"Feel it. A deep peace overcomes you. Your subconscious is registering all my words. You will obey. I am going to count to three . . . On three you will be incapable of saying your name. You will remember it, but you will no longer be able to speak it. One . . . Two . . . Three . . . See, you can no longer pronounce your name. Try it. You are incapable of doing so. Try again . . . The more you struggle, the less you succeed. Now you can no longer say your name."

THE SUBCONSCIOUS CANNOT BE FOOLED

It is possible to suggest to the person that he can no longer speak a given word. But let us return to the previous experiment. The candidate is unable to say his name. Nevertheless, he speaks fluently.

Certain people will start by saying the names of members of their family. For example:

"My mother's name is Mildred Miller. My brother is Alfred Miller. And I am . . ."

But from that point on, he will be blocked! The subconscious is not fooled by subterfuge . . . Even if the candidate has the same name, he will be unable to say it.

HOW DO YOU HEIGHTEN THIS SUGGESTION?

Here are the situations that show it is necessary to heighten the suggestion:

If, after some time has elapsed, the candidate begins saying his name again.

If the suggestion appears to be ineffective.

In both cases, the suggestion could take effect later on.

AND STILL MORE TESTS

Here are some more variations of suggestions to test his depth of hypnosis:

He cannot get up.

His finger becomes stuck to his nose.

However, as you get more and more training, you will not need this type of test. Straight off, you will perceive the depth of hypnosis. When you hypnotize a new patient, you will detect any change in behavior that shows he is coming out of hypnosis and will effectively mitigate it.

Volume III

Master Secrets of Undetectable Hypnosis On Others

EDITOR'S PREFACE

In this third volume of Prof. Tepperwein's system, "Secret Techniques of Hypnosis", you will encounter phenomena so surprising that your mind can scarcely conceive them: instant attraction of another person you have never met before, silent implantation of your thoughts in their mind, hypnosis by telephone, remote suggestion, hypnosis during sleep, and even walking on fire!

Not only will you discover them, but you will, for the most part, be given WORD FOR WORD what must be said to accomplish them yourself.

We must stress here the courage it took for Prof. Tepperwein to break the wall of silence surrounding these phenomena. In a century of narrow rationalism, to bear witness honestly to experiences like these may lead to outright blacklisting.

Prof. Tepperwein lifts the veil for you. He passes techniques on to you that, because of the astonishing power they bestow on those who master them, have been kept secret for centuries.

It is up to you to show yourself worthy of his trust. Do not yield to the intoxication of your new-found power. Use both restraint and wisdom throughout your apprenticeship and practice.

If the small amount of work that is required to master all these techniques momentarily discourages you, think of the benefits you will derive from them.

You will be able to help your children or your relatives eliminate their bad habits (incontinence, lack of attention in class, thumb-sucking, etc. for children; bulimia, tobacco, twitching, etc. for adults), without even holding a hypnotic session! Suggestions formulated during their sleep will be enough.

You will be able to create instant attraction for yourself in anyone you wish. You will even secretly and silently instill overwhelming sexual desire for you in those you choose.

You will be able to put a whole group of people under hypnosis — even skeptics — and accomplish what are presently unimaginable achievements.

You will be able to make a person do the bidding of your will, under your complete telepathic control, or induce hypnosis by means of a letter.

Once you are thus convinced of the Powers of the Mind — and therefore of your powers — you will possess total confidence in yourself. You will know that your fate is in your hands — that it is up to you to roll back the limits of the "possible" and achieve success, happiness and your full personal potential.

In fact, in putting this system at your disposal, this is the goal I seek to achieve. With all my wishes for your success, I remain your devoted,

Christian H. Godefroy,

Editor

SPECIAL HYPNOSES

HYPNOSIS BY TELEPHONE

THE CODE WORD

I have carried out numerous hypnotherapies over the telephone. The effects of this type of treatment are similar to the results obtained by direct hypnotherapy.

Have you already hypnotized the subject? By means of what suggestions? Pick up the one that has left its mark on the patient. It will serve as the "code word".

Implanted in the subconscious, this code word suggestion will trigger the hypnosis. And once he is under hypnosis, you can transform it into a post-hypnotic command.

Note: the distance between the patient and yourself will not influence the result. The subject to be treated should be assisted by a third person. Otherwise, under hypnosis, the receiver will slip from his hands and your contact will be broken.

Let me relate an incident which occurred during my first hypnotherapy by telephone:

The patient was no longer reacting to my words. No reply at the other end of the line. There was only one solution, to go to his home. I found him sleeping peacefully, the receiver hanging by his side. On awakening, he was surprised to see me and thought he was suffering from a hallucination.

As a result, I find it is preferable to have someone else present.

HOW TO AVOID THE PRESENCE OF A THIRD PERSON

It is preferable to have a third person present, but not indispensable. Suggest to the patient that he hold the receiver to his ear at all times. Insert this command several times among the suggestions on the course of treatment.

Once the subject is under hypnosis, heighten all suggestions save those which are the object of the hypnotherapy. But, above all, *the code word must be well established in his subconscious.*

AN EXAMPLE OF THE IMPLANTATION OF A CODE WORD

Have the patient visit you before initiating the hypnotherapy by telephone. Decide together on a code word. Once it is set firmly in the subconscious, it will automatically trigger the hypnosis.

Then, begin with the following suggestions (by telephone):

*"Put yourself at ease . . . Close your
eyes . . . They will remain closed
throughout our conversation . . .
Relax . . . Your arms and legs are
limp . . . Breathe deeply, slowly . . . Let
peace establish itself in you . . . Spread
throughout your body . . . Slacken your
muscles . . . Relax your nerves . . . Feel
it. You are quite calm . . . More and
more so . . . A pleasant weariness
envelops your body . . . You are sinking
more and more deeply into this feeling of
heaviness and weariness . . . Your whole
body is becoming heavier . . . More and
more . . . Your head, your eyelids are as
heavy as lead . . . Your eyes are tending
to close . . . You can hardly open
them . . . You no longer want to . . .
Surrender to this feeling of weariness
and heaviness . . . Your head and your
eyelids are heavier and heavier . . ."*

Once the patient is brought to this state, I begin
counting.

COUNTING WHILE INTERSPERSING LONGER AND LONGER PAUSES

I continue my suggestions:

"Soon, I will begin counting. At each number try to open your eyes, then close them again immediately ... Slowly ... You can hardly open your eyes ... Your eyelids grow heavier ... From one number to the next ... More and more ... I am counting. One, you can hardly open your eyes ... Two, your eyes grow heavier ... More and more ... Three, four ... Five, your eyelids are heavier and heavier ... Six ... Seven ..."

(Continue to count. Intersperse longer and longer silences. His eyes will close.)

THE SUGGESTION OF IMMOBILITY

Now, try other suggestions:

"Now, your eyes are hermetically closed. You can no longer open them ... You no longer want to ... Surrender to the beneficial feeling of weariness and heaviness ... Your body is growing heavier ... More and more ... Each finger is becoming as heavy as lead ... Feel how

*heavy and motionless your arms are . . .
Drawn towards the ground . . . More and
more . . . You can no longer lift them . . .
Try . . . You cannot do it . . ."*

Here is a variant of the suggestion.

THE SUGGESTION OF RELAXATION

*"You are quite calm . . . Relaxed . . . Don't
try to raise your arms any more . . . You
are sinking more and more deeply into
this wonderful feeling of weariness and
heaviness . . . Your whole body is as
heavy as lead . . . Feel it. You are more
and more tired . . . More and more . . . All
my words are registered in your subconscious . . . You will obey . . . You are experiencing a profound peace . . . All my
words are being definitely established in
your subconscious . . . If I say, KI-AI,
your eyes will close and you will fall
once more into this wonderful state of
peace and relaxation."*

(We have come to the code word)

THE CODE WORD: AN ABSOLUTE OBLIGATION

"If I say the word KI-AI, you will feel obliged to close your eyes . . . You will fall immediately into that pleasant state of relaxation and peace . . . It's obligatory . . . You will abide by it . . . The word KI-AI will be enough . . . You will close your eyes . . . You will surrender to the feeling of peace and relaxation . . . Absolute obligation . . . You will abide by it".

(Observe a minute of silence. The suggestions will have the time to register in the patient's subconscious. Strengthen them.)

"I am about to count to three . . . On three, stop concentrating . . . You will feel fresh and alert . . . But all my words are definitely implanted in your subconscious . . . You will abide by it . . . If I say the word KI-AI, your eyes close . . . You will fall once more into this beneficial state of peace and relaxation . . . Absolute obligation . . . You will abide by it . . . I now count to three . . . You will open your eyes . . . One-two-three: Open your eyes! Feel it. You are fresh

*and alert . . . Move your arms and
legs . . . Feel it. You are fresh and
alert . . . Fresh and alert."*

In this exercise, the word KI-AI, the code word, which has been deeply rooted in the patient's subconscious, will trigger the hypnosis. Repeat it several times under hypnosis. His eyes will close and he is under hypnosis.

INDUCE HYPNOSIS BY TELEPHONE

To induce hypnosis by telephone, I use the following words:

*"Please put yourself at ease . . . Breathe
slowly, regularly . . . I will soon say the
word . . . Your eyes will immediately
close, you will fall once more into this
beneficial state of peace and relaxation . . . As soon as I say the word, you
will feel obliged to close your eyes . . .
You will be under deep hypnosis . . . I
am saying the word KI-AI, KI-AI, KI-
AI".*

(As a safety measure, I repeat the word three times.)

"Now, your eyes are hermetically closed . . . You feel a deep peace . . . At each inhalation, you are sinking into an even deeper hypnotic state . . . Your hypnosis is deepening . . . At each inhalation . . . More and more . . . Your subconscious records all my words . . . They are etched into it . . . You will obey . . ."

Follow this with the desired suggestions, which are your goal.

HOW DO YOU INDUCE A FIRST HYPNOSIS BY TELEPHONE?

What are the necessary conditions? Experience and concentration.

If I have never seen the subject to be treated, I imagine him seated across from me. I address all my suggestions to this imaginary person who is listening to me on the telephone. A photograph of the patient will be a great help.

The percentage of success is very slightly below that of successes obtained by the practice of direct hypnotherapy.

HYPNOSIS INDUCED BY MEANS OF A TAPE RECORDER OR RECORD

A very widespread belief attaches to the following hypothesis: mysterious forces intervene under hypnosis. The hypnotist sets himself up as a magician, an enigmatic personage, the incarnation of the evil intentions of a higher spirit . . .

But, if hypnosis can be induced by simply listening to suggestions registered on cassettes or on a record, I ask you:

"Is this not proof that all these suggestions are erroneous, simplistic and absurd?"

Here is how it's done. The patient, lying on a couch, relaxes for a minute. He breathes slowly, regularly. He starts the equipment going, then concentrates on your voice.

These are your wishes and convictions that take effect. I have already explained it to you. I will prove it by the following examples.

EXAMPLE OF THIS TYPE OF HYPNOSIS

I record every hypnotherapy session on cassettes. The patient takes them away. In this way, he can resume treatment at will and deepen its effect.

Example: If the hypnotherapy proves effective, if he starts to stop smoking, or if he starts losing weight, record the suggestions that worked. Give the tape to him.

It is important that he play them several times every day. Since they are recorded with your voice, their content should be identified with your personality.

Patients who are difficult to hypnotize should listen to the cassettes all least three times a day. If the desired effect then begins to appear, have them return right away. Begin the hypnotherapy again at that point.

THE SIMPLICITY OF SELF-HYPNOSIS BY TAPE RECORDER

Make use of cassettes to achieve your own self-hypnosis. This is an invaluable aid.

Simply record your commands on cassette. Then let the effect of your voice take over.

HOW DO YOU RECOGNIZE THE CAUSE OF THE PATIENT'S PROBLEMS?

"Where do my difficulties come from?" This is a question you will often be asked.

Here is the way to discover the cause. First, the patient listens to a cassette on which the usual suggestions are recorded. Once the hypnosis is triggered, I tell him:

"I will say nothing for a few minutes. During this silence, you psychic eye will pick up the cause of your problems . . . You will provide an opening to your subconscious . . . This creates mental images of the cause . . . Now recognize the solution to your difficulties . . . And tell it to me".

If his subconscious does not immediately obey the command given, a repetition of the suggestions is essential. This allows you to avoid a long and costly treatment. The tape recorder will effectively replace you when you want it to.

Are the symbols that arise out of his first search into himself incomprehensible? Be reassured. *Repetition* will make images simpler and perfectly understandable.

LEARNING STIMULATED WITH THE HELP OF A TAPE RECORDER

Hypnotherapy stimulates schoolwork — and self-study for advancement in your career — in spectacular fashion. As a general rule, just one hypnotism will suffice. You will not only obtain an increase in the production of your schoolwork, but also the enthusiasm and skill of the true scholar for your work.

Record the following suggestions on tape and play them once a day.

If you are making this tape for yourself, use the word, "I", throughout. But if you are making the tape for someone else, use the word, "you" throughout.

"I am resting, calm, relaxed, my eyes closed. My arms and legs are flexible . . . I feel free, relaxed . . . Nothing distracts me . . . I let myself be drawn along . . . I am breathing slowly, regularly . . . I am quite relaxed . . . A wonderful peacefulness envelops my body.

"In this state of peace, I have an opening to my subconscious . . . This opening grows wider . . . More and more . . . My words are settling into my subconscious . . . Are taking root there . . . I will carry out these commands."

Let there be a brief pause.

"So far, I have been using only a small fraction of the true power of my mind . . . I have been using only 5 or 10 percent of the true power of my mind . . . Now I will begin to use more and more of it . . . Now I will begin to use it all.

*"When I need to learn something . . .
when I need to study . . . I will then automatically block all other thoughts
from my mind . . . My mind will be filled
only with what I need to learn . . . Everything else will disappear for that moment from my mind . . . I will think only
about what it is I have to learn . . . I will
open my mind to it like a great video
camera . . . I will automatically take all
of it in . . . I will automatically record it
on my memory like a video camera
records everything it sees and hears.*

*"I will think only about what it is I have
to learn . . . I will think about nothing
else . . . My full mind will be devoted to
taking it in . . . To recording it on my
memory . . . To be able to call it back to
my full mind anytime I wish . . . All my
memories will now become available to
me anytime I wish . . . All of them will be
ready to spring into my mind whenever I
need them . . . I can use all of them to
pass whatever tests life may give me . . .*

*To solve new problems . . . To create new,
winning ideas.*

*"I have the high-powered mind I have
always dreamed of . . . I can think now
with the best of them . . . I can learn
huge new vocabularies . . . I can now
memorize speeches, poems, sales presen-
tations, anything I need . . . I no longer
have to be ashamed of my mind or my
background or my memory . . . I can be
with the people I want to be with . . . I
can talk with them . . . I can make them
respect and listen to me and follow
me . . . I can have the mind I have always wanted . . . To give me the life I
have always wanted."*

HOW TO LIBERATE YOUR "BURIED GENIUS" OR THE GENIUS OF YOUR PATIENT

Record the following suggestions on tape, and play
them to yourself once a day. Or give the tape to the patient, and let him or her play it to themselves every day,
when necessary.

*"I am resting, calm, relaxed, my eyes
closed. My arms and legs are flexible . . .*

I feel free, relaxed . . . Nothing distracts me . . . I let myself be drawn along . . . I am breathing slowly, regularly . . . I am quite relaxed . . . A wonderful peacefulness envelops my body.

"In this state of peace, I have an opening to my subconscious . . . This opening grows wider . . . More and more . . . My words are settling into my subconscious . . . Are taking root there . . . I will carry out these commands."

Let there be a brief pause.

"For years, I have been using only my shallow, conscious mind . . . Now I will use all that mind, both conscious and unconscious . . . I will now draw on the vast storehouses of creativity in my unconscious mind . . . I will liberate the buried genius of that mind . . . I will see connections between ideas where I have never seen them before . . . I will build out of those new connections — one by one — new ideas that have never been thought of before . . . Profitable new

*ideas will now come easily to me ...
Beautiful words — phrases and sentences full of beautiful words — will
now come easily to me.*

*"My entire mind is now open to me ...
My entire memory is now open to me ...
Everything I have ever seen or heard is
now available to me ... I can explore all
this information at will ... Book after
book that I have read ... Magazine after
magazine that I have read ... Is waiting
in my mind to reveal its full details ...
To be combined with other details to
perfect new ideas.*

*"I can now control my dreams at will ...
I can tell my mind what to dream ... I
will only give my mind the beginning
and the direction of the dream ... And it
will go where it wants ... And it will
have that dream automatically give me
the answer to the problem I am
facing ... No matter what that problem
may be ... Whether it is a business or a
personal problem ... That dream will
give me the right answer."*

HYPNOSIS INDUCED BY MEANS OF A LETTER

THE WRITTEN WORD, CAPABLE OF TRIGGERING HYPNOSIS

Just like the code word, the written word can be implanted in the subconscious. Their effects are identical. It is important to choose a word not used in current language, the only way to avoid an accidental hypnosis.

I use the word KI-AI: a Japanese shout marking the beginning of a judo combat. It is not found in common language. For the method of implanting it in the subconscious, re-read the preceding text of this chapter.

NOTE: AN UNEXPECTED INCIDENT MAY ARISE

Here is one of these accidents:

I had two children of the same family under treatment, a boy of twelve and a girl of nine. I was to stimulate their schoolwork. But the family moved. How could the treatment be continued? I decided on hypnosis by letter. I set out the suggestions on paper. Here is the first part of it:

"Upon reading the word KI-AI, you will fall deeply under hypnosis. Your eyes remain open. Read the whole page. Ev-

*erything that follows will be registered
in your subconscious. Read this letter at
least once a day. You will faithfully
carry out the commands given".*

Everything seemed to work perfectly. The school results were very satisfactory. But, one day, I received a letter from the mother:

"I find myself obliged to put your letter under lock and key. Here is the reason. My daughter became aware that all she had to do was hold the beginning of your letter in front of her brother's eyes and he fell immediately under hypnosis. Then my daughter used his toys and things with impunity".

As a result, hypnosis induced by means of a letter presents unpleasant disadvantages. I have described it to you, so you can warn your patients of it.

INDIRECT HYPNOSIS

HOW TO INFLUENCE A PERSON WHO IS NOT HYPNOSENSITIVE

Here, the effective method is indirect hypnosis. Persons who are fundamentally not hypnosensitive are the mentally ill and introverted individuals who pay absentminded attention to the hypnotist.

"The Mysteries of Hypnosis" by Georges Dubois recounts all the hypnotherapies effected by Dr. Forbes, chief physician and founder of an insane asylum in London. 80,000 patients benefitted from his methods. He achieved extraordinary successes, beyond all expectations! He suppressed and cured mental illnesses, neuralgias and neuroses. When invited to an international congress, Dr. Forbes described his methods.

"One day, I was called to Milan, to the bedside of a lady of high society who was very ill. At that time I was staying near Turin. I took advantage of this to pay a visit to Lombroso. I spoke to him about my patient. He said that the subject was too introverted for the hypnotherapy to be effective.

"Only one solution was dictated. Indirect hypnosis or reflex hypnoses had to be applied."

HERE IS HOW INDIRECT HYPNOSIS IS DONE

The sick person is brought into the presence of a hypnotized subject. Then you proceed in the following order:

1. The patient, facing the subject under deep hypnosis, folds his arms. His right hand holds the

person's left hand. His left hand holds the
subject's right hand.

2. You address your suggestions exclusively to the
hypnotized subject.

3. The sick person, with his eyes open, attends the
treatment while fully conscious.

4. The hypnotized subject should detect the illness
of the patient. Deepen the hypnosis and then
ask him to describe the illness in detail.

5. The patient — through his contact with the person under hypnosis — transfers knowledge of
his illness to the hypnotized person. At the
same time, the person under hypnosis becomes
more and more similar to the sick person with
respect to his behavior, expressions and tone of
voice.

6. This shows that the transfer of personalities has
succeeded. Then you speak the suggestions for
relief, as we show you in the next volume.

7. Once the definitive suggestion for relief has
been spoken, the subject under hypnosis
awakens. Verify that the symptoms have
disappeared.

Question the intermediary subject. You will note that
no memory of the transfer of treatment or of illness re-

mains. The patient will be relieved of his ills a few days later.

Take this advice: *before ending the hypnosis, you must make sure that none of the transferred symptoms persist.*

ANOTHER FORM OF INDIRECT HYPNOSIS

The experiment was carried out by Dr. Alex. Just one hypnosensitive person is to be present at your office. The patient remains at home and relaxes to passively undergo the treatment. Of course you should set the time and duration of treatment by phone or mail.

What is the role of the medium — the hypnosensitive person who is in your office? He will undergo the hypnotherapy, receive the appropriate suggestions, and eventually have follow-up treatments if necessary.

TREATMENT FROM A DISTANCE

All the phenomena of the first experiment in indirect hypnosis are found here: the transfer of illness to the medium and the appearance of symptoms, etc.

Because of this, don't forget: before halting the hypnosis, remove all suggestions except those essential to effecting the cure.

Dr. Alex first controls the effects of treatment of the patient by telephone. He relieves the symptoms in the same way as you have been shown in the first indirect hypnosis experiment. He then waits a day or two to judge the depth of the patient's relief.

He then makes adjustments, if required.

Personally, though my experiments in this field are not conclusive, if I refer to my results, I dare to state that this treatment from a distance merits an in-depth study. It contains many very interesting and useful phenomena.

GROUP HYPNOSIS

The technique of group hypnosis differs very little from that of individual hypnosis. One condition must be observed: the room must be be calm and dark.

Avoid any dispersion of light, all possible noises in the immediate environment: slamming of doors, ringing of the telephone, etc.

Here is the difference between individual and group hypnosis. Group hypnosis always offers a chance of success. With individual hypnosis, not every case will inevitably be successful.

It is important to choose the participants with care. Each member of a group should possess the same potential for concentration, and the same quick reaction time.

How is group hypnosis triggered? Several techniques are adapted, the method of fixation in particular. Here is the procedure:

The participants concentrate on a blue bulb fixed to the ceiling or placed on a table. Then suggest that everyone cannot keep their eyes open. Then check that everyone has their eyes closed.

Only after this is accomplished do you give the appropriate suggestions.

WHAT IS THE IDEAL GROUP

The ideal group, made up of twelve or thirteen people, is easily controlled and directed. This restricted number allows the hypnotherapy to be applied to the participants while lying down.

With a number larger than this, from fifteen to fifty people, they must be seated. Here is how it's done.

Form rows of chairs, placing one behind the other. The first chair of each row remains unoccupied. Each person places his arms on the chair-back in front of him and puts his head on his arms.

Never go beyond fifty people. For numbers in excess of this number, you are practicing mass hypnosis, described in the following text.

SPIRITUAL CONTAGION WITHIN A GROUP

A current of sympathy and a spiritual contagion combine to stimulate this effect. Each person automatically puts himself at the spiritual level of the next and the result is a strengthening of sensations favorable to the carrying out of suggestions.

During this phenomenon, called "group spirit", a power superior to the total of all the hypnotic forces is working on each individual subject. Every member of this group should possess, at the same moment, the same degree of receptivity to the suggestions given.

I recommend that you improve the results achieved by group hypnosis in the following manner:

☐ first trigger a general hypnosis

☐ then give each individual a supplementary, individual suggestion.

THE ADVANTAGES OF GROUP HYPNOSIS

Here are the advantages: each person's suggestibilities are heightened by spiritual contagion — thus resulting in a saving of time. It is the perfect way to treat several people at once.

There is one drawback. A single member may shatter the contagion, and thus the result.

This is why it is a prime necessity to group psychically identical people together.

MASS SUGGESTION

FROM THE ISOLATED INDIVIDUAL TO A GROUP SPIRIT

The spiritual faculty of the "mass" is always superior to the sum total of the spiritual faculties of the individuals of which it is composed. The mass therefore reveals characteristics that do not exist in the isolated individual.

For example, self-awareness loses its importance here. Result: a collective spirit is created — a feeling of solidarity which directs personal will, imagination and feelings towards an objective that is common to the body of individuals.

Also, the reason for coming together soon becomes unimportant. None of the social reasons — profession, sex, environment, etc . . . have any more value.

The ideas which are dictated by the mass tend to become reality. The individual, isolated in the midst of this group, influenced by the superiority of numbers, acquires a force which urges him to obey its impulses and inclinations.

Primitive, potent inclinations — beyond all logic — are expressed. Once he is an integral part of the mass, he will perform actions he might never do alone. Outdoing oneself in good or evil can take on excessive proportions.

A FUSION THAT CREATES AN ACTIVE BEING

Once he is part of the mass, suggestion, like a spark, can be transformed into explosive action — and he will not even analyze its consequences.

In this situation, savagery, aggressiveness and enthusiasm create a new being. This characteristic is clearly demonstrated if all those assembled share the same religious convictions, similar political opinions, and an identical conception of the world. This, combined with spiritual outbursts, strengthens the effect of mass hypnosis on the single person.

HOW DO YOU ACHIEVE MASS HYPNOSIS?

The secret is simple, but incredibly powerful. You must present your own convictions in the form of mental images that are almost visible.

I repeat: the individuals that form the mass you are addressing or hypnotizing — every one of them — must be able to picture every detail of the mental image you are projecting.

They must be able to feel every emotion connected with that image, so each can reinforce the other's passion for it.

The spark of enthusiasm so created will ignite this mass. It will adopt the idea as its own. The general fervor will infect the most hesitant.

The idea will become reality.

HYPNOSIS IN THE WAKING STATE

Very receptive individuals will carry out suggestions in the waking state, if these are properly expressed. This hypnotic state — almost impossible to detect — is nonetheless a normal hypnosis. A correctly given suggestion will be sufficient to trigger this state.

How do you pick these people? Here is how it's done:

Hold out your hands to two persons in the audience — or to a new patient. Issue the command to take hold of your middle and index fingers. Suggest:

*"Hold my fingers tightly . . . Still
tighter . . . If I pull them . . . You can no
longer let go . . . Even away slowly . . .
Now, you can no longer let go . . . Follow
me".*

Gradually withdraw your hands. If the person lets go
of them, suggest:

"You can let go of my hand . . . Let it go".

In the contrary event, draw the subject along. Suggestion:

*"You can no longer draw your hand
away . . . Try it . . . You can no longer do
it . . . The more you try the less you will
let go . . . You are holding my hand
tightly".*

HYPNOSIS IN THE WAKING STATE AND THE POST-HYPNOTIC COMMAND

You can link a posthypnotic command to this type of
hypnosis. With the person already under hypnosis, suggest:

"Now, you will carry out all my commands in the waking state . . . You can-

*not, nor do you wish to do otherwise ...
Everything I command you to do, you
will obey in the waking state ...
Concentrate on my commands ...
Follow the numbers, one, two, three.
You will immediately carry them out ...
I am counting ... One ... Two ...
Three ... Nothing will prevent you from
obeying".*

These preparations finished, formulate a certain command. Count: one, two, three.

The subject submits!

LONG-DISTANCE HYPNOSIS

I would like to give you an example of hypnosis from a distance that is very much admired, but to most people is simply flabbergasting!

A FLABBERGASTING EXPERIMENT

Here is how it's done.

Address a group of people in these terms:

*"I am going into the next room. From
that place, I will oblige one of you to fall*

asleep. This phenomenon will be accomplished in one minute — thanks only to the intervention of my thoughts".

Select someone from the audience. Tell him:

"I am going into another room ... I will concentrate on you ... You will feel an irresistible need to sleep ... Fight it, your efforts will be in vain ... The more you resist, the quicker you will fall asleep ... At the end of one minute, you will be sleeping deeply".

Leave. At the end of one minute, return. The subject will in fact be sleeping!

It is recommended to choose an individual who has already undergone hypnosis: for example, a hypnosis in the waking state, carried out under your care. He will be more receptive to your command, since it will already be implanted in his subconscious. The simple fact of saying it will be enough to trigger the hypnosis.

How do you discover if the person is faking being hypnotized? Propose to the audience that they concentrate on achievable suggestions. You will transmit these to the subject under hypnosis, who absolutely must carry them out.

This experiment does not make use of true suggestion from a distance, but rather is a variation of hypnosis in the waking state.

HOW TO INFLUENCE HIM OR HER TO-WARDS A WELL-DEFINED GOAL

Having succeeded with the preceding experiment, formulate more complex commands.

Now try it with a group of people. It is necessary to mentally exclude one individual from this group. He will be useful in confusing any possible pretense.

It is essential to be convinced of your success. Doubt hinders the effect.

Next, begin suggesting the execution of the formulated command.

Here is an experiment opposite to the one above.

Put someone under hypnosis. Place yourself a few yards in front of him. Watch him. Concentrate. Say nothing, but think unceasingly:

"You will soon get up ... You will come towards me ... You will feel ill at ease ... There is nothing you can do

about it . . . Get up . . . Come to me with your eyes closed".

Then give the firm and brief command:

"Get up! Come!"

A profound spiritual contact will work an immediate effect. With a hesitant step, the person will rise and move in your direction.

Mentally direct him:

"Stop".

He will immediately come to a halt.

Here is how you discover any possible faking. Place yourself behind the person. Command:

"Fall backwards . . . Feel it. An irresistible force is pushing you . . . If you fall, I will hold you".

Your suggestions will be carried out.

CLASSIC EXPERIMENT OF FAMOUS MAGICIANS

Once you have arrived at an advanced level in the subject of hypnotism, try this classic experiment, performed by world-famous magicians.

Here is how it's done:

Put someone under deep hypnosis. Place him, eyes closed, with his back to the audience. Neither subject nor spectators can observe your movements.

Borrow some object from a member of the audience: his watch, for example. Slip it into someone else's pocket. Return to your person and turn him to face the audience. Direct him:

"You remain under deep hypnosis . . .
Open your eyes".

Add:

"A certain object can be found in the
pocket of a spectator . . . Go and find it
for me!"

Here is how to succeed with this experiment. Mentally steer the hypnotized subject towards the man dressed in a brown suit with the yellow tie. He is the one who has the object.

A further essential suggestion:

"Take the watch out of the left jacket pocket. Set your mind at rest, I am mentally supporting you".

The secret of success consists of mentally helping the person to discover the object in question. The result is guaranteed, if you effectively keep the subject under hypnosis. No one will attribute it to a collective illusion. No visible "trick" has been used. The supplementary and decisive mental suggestions remain unknown.

TO HELP CONCENTRATION

Hypnosis from a distance requires an "aid" to concentration. The simplest is a photograph of the subject to be hypnotized. Or you can picture the subject, seated facing you. Address your suggestions to this imaginary person.

Another way is to write your commands in a letter. Make a mental image of the patient receiving the mail, opening and reading it. Retain this distinct symbol for as long as possible. Banish doubt, which is an obstacle to success. (This letter will not really be sent, only in your imagination.)

HOW DO YOU DRAW YOUR THOUGHTS ALONG?

The Tibetan lamas and Indian gurus transmit their thoughts and commands to their followers, even if they have never seen them.

How do you achieve this true hypnosis from a distance, independent of the distance of the subject from you? The indispensable preparation is the sustained drawing along of your thought.

It is indispensable to properly master the technique of imagination. You psychic eye must conceive a precise mental image of the chosen object or event. And you must hold it there for as long as possible.

At home, practice this psychic concentration as much as possible. As your power strengthens, your results multiply.

Then try the following exercise.

THE TECHNIQUE OF IMAGINATION

Perform this experiment in a bus or train. Mentally select someone. Concentrate on that person. Think:

"You are becoming more and more tired . . . Your eyes are closing".

Create a mental image of the individual asleep. Your psychic eye will retain this symbol for a moment.

I advise you never to choose a child who is busy playing. Choose instead a traveler who is sitting quietly.

If the person closes his eyes, give these mental suggestions:

"Open your eyes . . . Feel that you are once more fresh and alert".

It is preferable not to look at the subject selected. Look in another direction or close your eyes.

EXPERIMENTS CARRIED OUT ON THE STREET

Concentrate on the nape of the neck of a passerby. Wish that he turn around . . .he will obey!

This classic phenomenon may be carried out at any time, if your strength of concentration exceeds all other sensory impressions which weaken it. It is a method of dominating a person.

Here is a variation. Concentrate on the nape of an individual's neck. Make a mental image of the following actions: he pauses before a store window, he buys some ice cream or a certain newspaper, etc . . . As a general rule, he will carry out your commands.

Depending on your psychic form, you may have more or less success on different days. I urge you to intensify your trainings. *Develop your gifts without respite.*

ENFORCED WILL AND PERSONAL DECISION

The will and personal decision are relative. We all know that every day we carry out behavior imposed by unconscious decisions.

Say to an individual whom you have hypnotized, and to whom you have suggested a certain action:

"You are buying an ice cream at this very moment that I have commanded you to do it".

He will offer you a reason that is quite plausible, and will energetically deny having been the object of your decision.

We have conditioned the behavior of individuals by electrical stimulation of certain parts of the brain. They carried out what the stimulation made them do. But *they still maintained that their actions were due to their own decision.*

To sum up: choose a certain behavior. Transmit it to an individual. *He will always be convinced of having decided on it himself.*

THE EXPERIMENT OF DR.DUSART

In the book of Dr. Richard Baerwald, *Die Intellektuellen Phänomene,* Dr. Dusart reports:

"Every day I went to see a certain Miss L.; I would leave upon privately giving her the command to awaken at a certain time on the following day. One day I omitted my suggestion. I remembered it on my way, half a mile from her home. The idea came to me to give the command from this distance. I formulated: You will sleep until eight in the morning.

"Next day, I arrived shortly before eight at the home of my sleeping (hypnotic sleep) client. To the question, 'Why are you still asleep at this hour?', I received the reply, 'But, doctor, I am carrying out your command!' I retorted, 'You are mistaken. Yesterday, I did not command you to sleep.' Reply: 'Certainly. But, five minutes after you left, I heard you tell me, 'Sleep. You will awaken at eight in the morning!' "

"It was now eight o'clock. The following fears nagged at me:

"Would habit not generate an illusion of the senses?

"Would the reaction not be the result of chance?"

"To reassure my professional conscience and to eliminate my doubts, I directed the patient, 'Continue sleeping. I will wake you'.

"During that day, I had a free quarter of an hour. I decided to go and check on my patient. I left my quarters, five miles from her home. As I left, I thought, 'Wake up!', with a glance at my watch. Two o'clock.

"Arriving at my patient's home, I found her awake. At my injunction, her parents had noted the hour she awoke: two o'clock! I repeated the experiment several times with identical results."

This report was published on May 16, 1875 in the "Medical Tribune". The technique of hypnosis from a distance is therefore not a novelty. The only difficulty is to train the faculty of concentration and the power of imagination.

Persist, persevere.

HOW TO READ ANOTHER PERSON'S THOUGHTS WITHOUT THEIR SAYING A WORD.

Now let us concern ourselves with more practical, everyday applications of this hypnosis-at-a-distance:

Let us say that you meet an attractive person of the opposite sex at a party — or a person important to you at a business meeting. As you know, the chances of becoming intimately acquainted with that person's thoughts.

during this first meeting, are practically non-existent. But hypnosis can perform the breakthrough you desire.

First you must make eye-contact with this person. If you are introduced to him or her, that will be sufficient. If not, go up to that person and introduce yourself. Even if you are dismissed, the necessary eye-contact has been established.

During that eye-contact, think (but do not say aloud) the following words:

"I am now opening your mind to me . . . I will do you no harm . . . But, from this moment on, your mind will be open to me".

That is all that is necessary to gain entry. Then leave this person, and go to a quiet corner of the room.

When you established eye-contact, you commanded your mind to make a mental photograph of that person's face. You commanded your eyes to search out every feature of that person's face and body. Now, when you are standing alone, you close your eyes — or stare at a blank wall in the room — and recreate a mental picture of that person, so vividly that you could almost reach out and touch him or her.

Now you put yourself into a state of instant deep self-hypnosis — as shown in volume 4 of this set — by saying the following words, which you have previously memorized:

"I am penetrating deep into my unconscious mind . . . I have at my command all the powers of my unconscious mind . . . I am able to send my mind across space and time".

NOW THE OTHER PERSON'S THOUGHTS COME POURING OUT TO YOU

Keep the other person's face clearly before you in your imagination. And then think these words:

"You will now whisper to me your thoughts . . . You will whisper what you are thinking to me at this moment".

It is imperative that you use the word, "whisper", in this command, since it carries with it the idea of secret sharing. Now listen carefully. Even if the room is crowded and noisy, within this noise you will slowly begin to hear the distinct whisper of this chosen person's thoughts.

You cannot yet direct these thoughts, but you can eavesdrop on them. Do not be confused if they are not phrased in full sentences, as ordinary conversation is. They are more likely to be reactions: a few words here and there, some of which make sense to you and some of which do not.

They will also carry strong emotions — uncensored emotions. For the other person has no need to disguise them, or make them polite. You will feel the emotions as clearly as you will hear the words.

(You must remember, the first time you conduct such an experiment, you will not get full entry into that other person's mind. You will get only flashes of her or his thoughts. The ability to hear them all is a hypnotic skill, which must be practiced again and again, until it is strengthened and then mastered.)

Now, once you have established contact with the other person's thoughts, move into his or her line of sight. Perhaps pass closely by, and smile. This simple action will bring you back into his or her thoughts. But this time you are receiving those thoughts. Now you are in a position to know the truth about what he or she really thinks about you. Information that otherwise would, at best, be given to you only months from now, or, at worst, never given to you, is now yours at once.

No matter how good or bad those thoughts are, you are now ready to go on and begin implanting telapathic suggestion into that other person's mind.

VITAL NOTE:

The primary law of hypnosis — to state it once again — is this: It can not be effectively used to make someone do ANY ACT or feel ANY EMOTION that would HARM them. This applies to secret hypnosis as well as declared hypnosis.

Therefore, what you are now going to suggest must be as good for him or her as it is for you. If you are going to build overwhelming sexual attraction, for example, you must realize that this is nothing more than ATTRAC-TION . . . nothing more than a willingness to first get to know you better, and then want to try the beginning steps towards sexual union.

By no means will this secret hypnosis — nor any other means of hypnosis — turn this other person into your "sexual slave", or other such absurd fantasies. Nor will you be able to "pervert" this other person's feelings into entering into any other social, monetary or business relation with you that is against his or her better interests.

Hypnosis is a tool for gaining what is rightfully yours, as well as what is rightfully the other person's. It is a shortcut for making possible what, without it, would never be possible. Right now, you know very well that you deserve far more from life than what it has so far given you. When you see the person to whom you are sexually attracted, for example, you know, in your heart of hearts, that it would be good and right for that person to be just as powerfully attracted to you. You know that you could make that person happy.

But today, for whatever reasons of fate are now blocking you, YOU DO NOT HAVE THAT CHANCE. Secret hypnosis gives you a powerful tool for correcting that. It enables you to do what should have been done. It makes possible what will be best for both of you. This is the key. What is best for both of you. Follow that rule, and you will be a master of hypnosis . . . and of fate.

HOW TO CREATE INSTANT ATTRACTION AND EVEN OVERWHELMING SEXUAL DESIRE THROUGH THIS SECRET HYPNOSIS.

You have now gained entry to the other person's mind. His or her thoughts flow out to you. Now you are to start influencing those thoughts.

This can be done either when you are in the presence of this person, or even when you are far apart from him or her. The essential element is not how close you are, but how powerful your hypnotic concentration is.

If you are alone, close your eyes, and throw every other thought out of your mind. If you are in the same room, stare at that person — even behind his or her back — until you can see nothing else in the room but that one person. Until there is no one in that room for you but that one person.

Now think these thoughts:

"Your mind is now opening to me ... I am entering your thoughts ... What I am thinking, you will now begin to think".

(Memorize these words carefully. Repeat them over and over again. Practice filling them with all the new emotional power hypnosis has given you. Devote 15 minutes a day for a week to them. Feel the magnetism in them rise with each new practice session. Feel the conviction in them grow until it becomes overwhelming.)

Now, if you are creating active interest in someone for business purposes, think something like this. The exact words are not necessary, only the general structure of the ideas are.

"I am, without your knowledge, focusing your mind ... This gentle focusing will open up new worlds of opportunity to you ... Think of (give your own name) ... Who is he? ... What is it about him that is so impressive? ... Could he be of help in the problems you are facing? ... You have a feeling that he

may be the answer ... That he may be the solution ... Something inside you — deep inside you — cannot let the thought of him go ... You must find out more about contact with him."

Or, if you are creating a wanted decision in someone, think something like this. The exact words are not necessary, only the general structure of the ideas are.

"I am, without your knowledge, focusing your mind ... This gentle focusing will open up new worlds of opportunity to you ... Think of (give your own name) ... What did she recently tell you? ... Why did you not realize how perceptive her insights were? ... Why did you dismiss what she said? Why did you not act on what she said? ... You have a feeling that she may have the answer ... That she may have the solution ... Something inside you — deep inside you — cannot leave what she said go ... You must find out more about it from her ... Right now, get in contact with her."

Or, if you are creating fervent sexual desire in someone for you, think something like this. The exact words are not necessary, only the general structure of the ideas are.

"I am, without your knowledge, focusing your mind ... This gentle focusing will open up new worlds of love and happiness and fulfillment to you ... Think of (give your own name) ... At first you thought he was not attractive ... But as you look back on your meeting with him now, you realize that you overlooked SO MUCH in him ... Think of his eyes ... They were so deep and so compelling ... And the gentleness and the power you sensed deep within him.

"Think of his hands ... They were so strong ... What would it feel like to be sheltered by those hands? ... to be touched by those hands?

"You have a feeling ... A strange, deep feeling ... That he may be the answer ... That he may be what you have been looking for all your life ... That he may open up the true you ... That he may let you reach down deep inside yourself and

*touch true passion . . . Something inside
you — deep inside you — cannot leave
this feeling of wanting him . . . Of wanting to see him again . . . Of wanting to
talk to him again . . . Of wanting to
touch and touch and touch him . . . You
must locate him again . . . Right now,
you must — you simply must — get in
contact with him again."*

With these tools of secret hypnosis at your command,
you will take charge instead of submit, lead instead of follow. You will have decisive influence on others. Status
and power will be delegated to you. Success will smile and
destiny will bow to your superior concentration and in-
flexible willpower.

Before to know it, you will find yourself endowed with
the power of authority over everyone you encounter.
Practice. Practice. Practice. Think of a tomorrow when
you have psychic, secret, invisible influence on others.

HOW TO SURROUND YOUR BODY WITH AN INVISIBLE FIELD OF PHYSICAL MAGNETISM

Record the following suggestions on tape, and play
them to yourself once a day:

"I am resting, calm, relaxed, my eyes closed. My arms and legs are flexible . . . I feel free, relaxed . . . Nothing distracts me . . . I let myself be drawn along . . . I am breathing slowly, regularly . . . I am quite relaxed . . . A wonderful peacefulness envelops my body.

"In this state of peace, I have an opening to my subconscious . . .This opening grows wider . . . More and more . . . My words are settling into my subconscious . . . Are taking root there . . . I will carry out these commands.

"I am now reaching into every cell of my body . . . Every cell, from the top of my head, to my face, to my shoulders, to my chest, to my abdomen . . . To my pelvis, to my legs, to the bottom of my feet . . . Every cell, in every part of my body, has now risen to a higher state of power . . . Is glowing like a high-energy dynamo . . . Is giving off magnetism that turns others irresistibly towards me . . . That pulls what I want and what I need out of my surroundings.

"My body is now surrounded by this invisible field of physical magnetism . . . It never tires . . . It never dims . . . It is always there to protect me . . . To draw to me what I want . . . "

Let there be a brief pause.

"From this moment on, I will be rid at last of my inhibitions and my destructive emotions and my insecurities . . . Why should I continue them when I have this magnetic power at my bidding? . . . Instead, I will now have the power to fascinate someone by a single look, or by nothing more than the tone of my voice . . . In every romantic relationship I choose, the other person will want me every bit as much as I want them.

"I am now in constant touch with this subconscious dynamo . . . I command this physical magnetism . . . My former bad habits fade away under its power . . . I have the self-confidence I have always dreamed of . . . I can now make my dreams become my realities . . . I have the power to do this . . . I will use this power wisely . . . It will help others

at the same time it helps me . . . I will do no harm with it . . . It is too great to misuse . . . I will employ it for good only . . . For my good . . . And for the good of the world."

DRUG-INDUCED HYPNOSIS

Certain narcotics induce hypnosis. They are to be used not to anesthetize the patient, but to produce perfect relaxation.

Inject small doses slowly, regularly, to avoid a possible loss of consciousness. Your goal is to restrict the field of consciousness, to increase the suggestibility of the subject and to eliminate obstacles due to conscious inhibitions.

APPROPRIATE MEDICATION

Every therapist selects "his" narcotic from an existing range. O. Wetterstrand and Krafft-Ebing are satisfied with the effects obtained thanks to chloroform. Moll prefers chloral hydrate. Schupp uses ethylene bromide. A brief intoxication due to chlorethylene will encourage the triggering of hypnosis.

One medication is very effective: it is paraldehyde, a sedative and hypnotic. The normal dose is from three to five grams. The single maximum dose is five grams. The daily maximum should be no more than ten grams.*

*Pascal Brotteaux, and subsequently Prof. Henri Baruk, used scopochloralose with success: in a medium dosage, 0.50 mg. scopolamine and 0.50 chloralose (light trance) or in a heavy dosage, 0.75 mg. scopolamine and 0.75 chloralose (hypnosis) — the chloralose must be absolutely pure and thoroughly mixed in the tablet. Ref. *L'hypnose*, Prof. Henri Baruk, ed. P.U.F. 1974 (N.D.E.)

PRACTICE RESERVED EXCLUSIVELY TO DOCTORS

This text is addressed solely to the reader who is a physician. Its motive is to induce hypnagogic relaxation by means of medication.

Here is an inoffensive but effective stimulant: a mixture of three volumes of carbonic acid and seven volumes of oxygen. The inhalation of the resultant carbonic gas induces light hypnosis and certain psychic changes which increase the suggestibility of the subject.

POST-HYPNOSIS

Definition: This is a suggestion that you give to your patient under hypnosis — which he later executes at a precise moment after you have restored him to the waking state.

Here is how it's achieved:

While he is in hypnosis, you give him the command. Although he shows no reaction at that instant, the command is recorded in his unconscious.

What you have done is this: You have conditioned his subconscious to carry out that command at a given moment, when he is outside the hypnotic state.

In one of my cases, between one and two years went by before the suggestion was carried out!

I will now quote a classic example reported by Professor Bernheim.

CLASSIC CASE

It was August. I had commanded Sergeant-Major S. under hypnosis:

> *"Listen! On the first thursday of October, you will go to the residence of Dr. Liébeault. There you will meet the President of the Republic who will award you a decoration".*

I met Sergeant S. several times. Neither he nor I mentioned the posthypnotic command. On Thursday, October 3rd — sixty-three days after this command — I received a letter from Dr.Liébeault:

"Today, at 1:10 P.M., S. burst into my home. Without paying any attention to those present, he went directly to the bookshelves. There, I watched him. He bowed respectfully and said, 'Your Excellency'. He then held out his hand and said, 'Thank you, your Excellency'."

To the question, "To whom are you talking?" he replied, "To the President of the Republic, of course." Yet another bow; then he went away.

Mr. F., a witness to this scene, questioned me concerning this "madman". I retorted, "Mr. S. is as normal as you or I".

You must be aware that posthypnotized persons are unaware of the motivation for their actions (the posthypnotic command), and that they are firmly convinced of their freedom of decision. They will deny any suggestion that you have interfered with their own free will.

EXPERIMENT CARRIED OUT WITH THREE PEOPLE

The psychologist H.E. Hammerschlag, a leading light on the subject of hypnosis, reports a case of post-hypnosis carried out on three people at the same time.

To subject A., he gave the suggestion:

"Upon awakening, you will move the inkwell from my desk to the window-sill".

To subject B., he suggests:

"Upon awakening, you will put the chair, that is placed near the window, upon my desk".

To subject C., he suggests:

"Upon awakening, you will stick out your tongue at me at the first word I utter".

Here are the results:

A. Awakens. Sits beside the desk; steals a glance at the inkwell, visibly ill at ease. Suddenly he rises, seizes the object, puts it on the window-sill.

B. Awakens. Refuses to sit on the chair placed near the window; tensely observes the hypnotist's gestures, who pretends to set an object to rights, and turns away. Immediately, B. sets the chair on the hypnotist's desk. When asked, "Why did you do that?", he answers, "It's a joke".

C. Seated facing the hypnotist. Talks about his well-being, a tense expression on his face. He appears to be resisting an idea which is forcing itself upon him. I ask, "What idea just crossed your mind?" Ashamed, he admits, "I wanted to stick out my tongue at you".

This experiment bears out the theory: the posthypnotic command is carried out in the waking state. I should say "seems" to be executed in this state. For my experiments have repeatedly proved the following fact: before carrying out the command, the subject falls once more under a very brief hypnosis, broken by accomplishing the posthypnotic action.

Let us consider the example of C. His refusal to carry out the command is quite normal. In this case, principles and upbringing won out over the suggestion. This proves: *suggestions contrary to fundamental personality inclinations are automatically cancelled.*

BEHAVIOR OF THE PATIENT

How does a hypnotized subject behave during the time between ending the hypnosis and the moment of carrying out of the posthypnotic command? Normally.

No memory of the suggestion appears to persist.

But, once the moment arrives, the memory of this command and a growing compulsion to obey operate strongly on the subject. If he is free of any inhibition, he will carry it out without hesitation.

You may give a supplementary suggestion.

"The action accomplished at the time determined seems to be done of your own free will. Any suggestion is erased from your memory."

Note: You may have to repeat the posthypnotic suggestions several times. At what moment will the patient obey the command given? You should count on a delay of three to four hours.

A SAFETY PRECAUTION FOR THE HYPNOTIZED SUBJECT

The patient's subconscious will block any posthypnotic suggestion from his memory. This may be dangerous for him, so I recommend: *never forbid the recollection of a post-hypnotic command.*

However, you may reverse the order given at any time if it is inconvenient.

Incidently, if you suggest an immoral action, the patient's subconscious will transmit it to the censorship of the conscious mind.

Is the subject aware of an acceptable posthypnotic command? Be reassured, he will not be aware. And he will obey, for the suggestion is implanted within the range of his allowed actions.

We now reveal the following law:

If the will and feelings are opposed, the latter will prevail.

Here is an example:

A SPECIAL EXPERIMENT

The famous American psychologist, G.H. Estabrooks, an expert on the subject of hypnosis, suggested to someone:

"At a given signal, you will go to the window. See the pack of cards on the window-sill. Remove the ace of spades. Give it to me".

The hypnotized subject was a student of psychology, very knowledgeable in the subject of hypnotism. The result was as follows:

He went to the window, took the pack of cards, turned and said,

"I am convinced that this is a posthypnotic command!"

"And what do you intend to do?" asked the hypnotist.

"I want to take the pack of cards and give you the ace of spades."

"Correct. It is in fact a posthypnotic suggestion. And now?"

"I will not carry out the command."

"Good. But I will make a bet with you: you won't be able to stop yourself from doing it."

"You're on!"

THE POWER OF POST-HYPNOTIC INFLUENCE

The result was very interesting. Two hours passed. From time to time, the subject went to the window, came back, distressed, convinced of being unable to comply. At the end of two hours, the professor declared: "You have won the bet!"

But, that very afternoon, a peculiar things happened. The power of the posthypnotic command plagued the student. The obligation to obey became a torment, a fixation. He came back to the hypnotist's house, and carried out the command.

This experiment shows that *the power of posthypnotic influence on the subconscious of a normal, healthy person is immeasurable.*

In medicine, this posthypnotic command is the essential part of hypnosis. It is this that governs the significant effects of a therapy: to suppress or cure an illness, or to change inappropriate behavior.

HOW TO HYPNOTIZE THE PATIENT DURING SLEEP

A PATH LEADING DIRECTLY TO THE SUBCONSCIOUS

What is hypnosis during sleep? It is the method of hypnotizing another person in spite of his wishes.

It is also the path leading directly to his subconscious. The criticism and doubt of the conscious mind are nonexistent when the subject is asleep.

What are the favorable times?

They are the first two hours of sleep, and the hour before awakening.

ESTABLISH RAPPORT

First, establish rapport — contact between yourself and the subconscious of the sleeping person. Here is how it's done.

As soon as you enter the room, start speaking gently to him — but only in this way:

Come to within three feet of the sleeping subject. Address your suggestions to him while looking at the pit of his stomach. Never speak his first name, he would awaken.

Stationed near the door, whisper these suggestions:

"Do not be disturbed . . . Continue sleeping . . . Your sleep is getting deeper and deeper . . . More and more . . . Nothing disturbs you . . . You are feeling quite well . . . Your sleep is becoming deeper and deeper . . . Now, you are in deep sleep, but you can hear me".

THE DESIRE TO HELP

Be careful to avoid any effort of selfishness on your part. Your only motivation must be to aid the individual.

Note that this tender concern works towards a very satisfying result. A feeling of peace and harmony — in both him and you — will result.

What are the risks? This question is often put to me by anxious parents. My reply: none.

I explain: a suggestion that is inappropriate to the situation can be immediately replaced by another that is in opposition to the first.

This type of hypnosis is particularly suited to eliminating certain defects and shortcomings of children such as the refusal of any food, bedwetting or disastrous school results. A rapid result is guaranteed.

FORMULATE POSITIVE SUGGESTIONS

Avoid negative turns of phrase.

Do not say, "You will not wet your bed any more," but, "From now on, you will wake up, go to the toilet and go right back to sleep".

Do not suggest, "You do not have a headache anymore," but, "Your head is now free of any hurt".

Do not state, "You will not refuse to eat any longer!" but, "You will be glad to be able to eat. You will have a good appetite".

Doctor Alfred Brauchle reports in his book, *Hypnose und Autosuggestion* (Reclam, 1961):

For years, a middle-aged patient suffered regular occurrences of heart failure. All medical treatment proved ineffective. In four weeks, his wife cured him with the help of suggestions regularly repeated during his sleep.

Here is another example:

The son of a friend, five years of age, sucked his thumb. Rewards, punishments, nothing worked. A single firm suggestion, given by his father during sleep, immediately resolved the problem.

Stuttering, incontinent children — or those afflicted with most other ailments — will be cured by this type of hypnotherapy.

AN EXAMPLE:

Fritz Lambert relates:

"A woman who came before my committee made the following report:

'I applied the suggestion while my husband was asleep. For a very long time, he had not been digesting certain foods. Three hypnotherapies were enough to cure him' ".

If a single suggestion, repeated three times, had been enough to eliminate an ailment of very long standing, an accurate idea can be formed of the real power of this type of hypnosis.

RESPECTING THE WISHES OF THE SLEEPING PERSON

Hypnosis from sleep will convince the most hardened skeptics.

Here is the principle of your success: Be sure of yourself. Have no doubts about the effect of your suggestions. Dispel any fear of the possible awakening of the sleeping person. The transfer of such feelings could be prejudicial to the basic objective.

Do not directly suppress reprehensible behavior by an outright command. Instead, make the person to be treated *want to change* a deplorable habit or a personal defect. Example:

For example, do not directly command:

"From this moment, you will not smoke".

Instead say:

"You no longer experience any more interest in smoking".

Remember: If you directly block a behavior — and, at the same time allow the desire for it to remain in the patient's subconscious — that desire will eventually prevail.

So do not suggest:

"You will not drink anymore".

Say instead:

"You have lost all desire to drink".

Remove the desire first, and the behavior will disappear along with it.

Or to put it another way: If the blocked behavior and the desire for it neutralize each other, there will be no result.

What happens if the hypnotherapy during sleep does not take immediate effect? Never fear. You have poorly established rapport or contact. In no way be discouraged, but proceed in another fashion. Reinforce your original suggestions in this way:

"Continue to sleep deeply ... You will now hear my words more distinctly ... You will answer the following questions without re-awakening".

Next, question the sleeping person:

"Sleep deeply: Can you hear me?"

With the first yes, be reassured. Your suggestions are registering in the subconscious, your commands will be carried out.

"IMPOSSIBLE ACCOMPLISHMENTS" DURING SLEEP

Examples:

A famous model lost thirty pounds in three months by simple suggestive therapy during sleep.

A television producer learned the most difficult language in the world in ten days — mandarin Chinese. It was possible for him to hold a conversation with a Chinese consul.

How had he accomplished this feat? By recording different lessons on endless cassettes which ran at night while he slept.

This procedure is also used to achieve other desires — correction of a shortcoming, stimulation of schoolwork, and the improvement of professional or sporting performances.

HYPNOSIS BY WHISPERING

INCREASE IN ATTENTION

Is someone whispering about you? At once, your attention is applied to following this conversation. Make use of this reaction to concentrate someone's attention on your words.

To prove this, draw someone into a conversation. Lower your voice imperceptibly. More and more. Your interlocutor will automatically adjust to the range of your voice. You will both end up by whispering.

Then I ask the person:

"Why are you whispering?"

I get no explanation in reply. Only at this precise moment does my companion become aware of the very low tone of the conversation.

A TYPE OF HYPNOSIS ESPECIALLY BENEFICIAL TO NERVOUS PEOPLE

If you attempt to induce hypnosis by the usual methods on nervous, anxious people, this will be impossible to accomplish. But reassuring suggestions, spoken in a very low monotone, will trigger the hypnosis.

Here is how it is done:

With the patient lying comfortably, eyes open, begin by addressing appropriate suggestions to him so as to create a climate of trust and relaxation. Your tone will be normal.

Lower it progressively. The patient will whisper, then he will close his eyes.

If this does not happen, suggest:

"Now, close your eyes . . . With each breath, you are sinking still more into a pleasant feeling of peace and relaxation".

Then, return to the usual words. Whisper them. Once the hypnosis is triggered, slowly raise your tone to normal.

HYPNOSIS IN SUCCESSION

THE CONTACT

In hypnosis in succession, forces appear which are similar to those which arise in group hypnosis. The powers are strengthened by mutual contact of the participants.

How do you start? Six persons, seated with eyes closed, hold hands and form a circle. You can then give them a great feeling of peace and relaxation, which can be deepened by oral suggestions.

EXAMPLE

One day I set up a sequence with five skeptics and only one hypnosensitive individual. The enormous difference between the forces present caused me to try to postpone the session. But the patients decided against that. Here is what took place:

By appropriate suggestions, I put the patient susceptible to influence under hypnosis, to the surprise of the five other participants, who stealthily kept an eye on one another's reactions.

But, here is the incredible part. The transfer of the hypnotic effect of a single person had succeeded in putting the five others under hypnosis . . . in eight minutes! How can it be explained?

Professor Matthias of Zurich wrote on the subject:

"The vegetative and spiritual life of the human being cannot be maintained in activity without an electrophysiological bipolarity: the cations and the anions. This biological process rests on electronic phenomena tied to atoms".

As a result, it will involve a permanent exchange of negative and positive forces, conditioned by the constant process of charge and discharge of each cell of the organism.

THE SYNCHRONIZATION OF FORCES

We must acknowledge the following reality: contact among several people creates a blending of these forces. They can shift either to the positive or the negative side of one of the participants. But the forces which take precedence will certainly be felt by the others in the group.

Note that a single skeptical participant can prevent a patient susceptible to influence from falling into a hypnotic state. Keep this in mind during your practice.

HYPNOSIS THROUGH MAGNETISM

WHAT IS MAGNETISM?

By definition, magnetism is the sum of the energies of concentration of matter. Do not confuse animal magnetism, the influence of one person over another, with the magnetism that attracts certain metals to each other.

By magnetism, I mean the effect of the exchange of positive and negative forces, produced by the charge and discharge of each cell of the organism.

This type of magnetism exists to a greater or lesser degree in every living being.

Discover it. Subject it to your will. Make use of it at your pleasure.

NO BODY WITHOUT MAGNETISM

Magnetism exerts a molecular attraction. Atoms and molecules, collected in great number in our bodies, make up our original substance. Through its attracting effect, magnetism brings them together in one form: the body.

Its externalization by any natural movement is called irradiation, or attraction of one person for another.

CAUTION: The magnetic influence of one human being can dominate the will of another, even to the total submission of the latter. But the subjugated individual will not willingly agree to this.

POSITIVE OR NEGATIVE IRRADIATION

We find this type of magnetism in animal and plant life.

An example of positive irradiation:

Approach to within about three of four yards of a fine and ancient tree. You will be placed on its line of force. Let yourself be surrounded by its irradiation; you will "recharge" yourself if your "battery" is dead.

EXAMPLE OF NEGATIVE IRRADIATION

The opposite phenomenon may take place. You have already had the experience of distinctly feeling an obvious antipathy for a human being you have hardly met. His irradiation was in disharmony with your magnetism.

THE ADDITION OF FORCES

Gather together a large number of people.

The sum of radiant magnetism represented by each person creates a certain force. This force absorbs individuality. Each of us will submit to the same single force. We will be "part" of the mob.

If you had this experience, *it will take days for you to rid yourself of this invisible bond, of its influence.*

We deduce that every body possesses a biological irradiation. Certain human beings have a very large measure of it. This power allows them to preserve the lives of small animals and plants.

If you do not as yet possess this gift, don't be downhearted. At this very moment, magnetism is enough of an integral part of you to induce hypnosis.

In an old volume, I discovered a special healing magnetic treatment.

HOW IS HEALING HYPNOSIS TRIGGERED BY SPECIAL MAGNETIC TREATMENT?

The ill patient is seated comfortably on a chair, eyes closed. His feet are on the floor, his hands placed on his thighs.

The magnetizer, erect or seated before the patient, concentrates his attention on the relief to be attained. Then, he magnetizes the sick person.

He uses circular magnetic passes, with his fingers slightly folded towards the palm. The passes finished, the healer shakes his hands. This movement is necessary to eliminate the germs of the illness.

The procedure is repeated several times. The sick person experiences a great feeling of well-being.

Or the magnetizer begins by the laying on of hands. For example, the right hands on the right shoulder of the patient, and his left hand on the patient's left shoulder. The magnetic current will pass through the body of the patient from the right hand to the left of the operator.

We deduce from this that the patient's body is the resistance to the magnetic current. The healer will feel a slight tingling in his hands.

Another way of going about it. The magnetizer places his right hand on the solar plexus, his left on the back of the patient's head. The positive hand (right hand), will preferably be in direct contact with the skin of the pit of the stomach.

If the patient is not to be unclothed, the magnetizer will leave his hand for some time on this clothed part. The magnetic force will spread throughout the body from the solar plexus, from the head to the feet. A salutary fluid will envelop the patient: he will feel either cold or heat.

It is not absolutely necessary to touch the body during the passes. Hypersensitive people often achieve a state comparable to deep hypnosis. Their psychic activities are found to be clearly improved.

INCREASE OF SENSITIVITY

A person showing hypersensitivity — that is, a person who you have discovered is especially suggestive — is favorable for your first hypnosis. In this hypnotic state, *the posthypnotic command will encourage another deeper hypnosis.*

SPLIT HYPNOSIS

This procedure, perfected at the turn of this century by A. Vogt, stamps out all problems you may encounter. Here is how it is applied:

Begin by inducing the hypnosis by a method of your choosing. Then split it. By this I mean that, from time to time, you bring the patient out of his hypnotic state, and question him concerning his impressions and reactions. In this way, you will disclose what part of your system suits him and what other part proves upsetting.

In this way, you adapt your procedure to the reactions of the patient.

EXAMPLE

Here is an example. Let us suppose that you have induced a first hypnosis in these terms:

"Put yourself at ease ... Slacken the muscles of your arms and legs ... Relax ... Breathe slowly, regularly ... At each inhalation, you sink deeply into a pleasant feeling of peace and relaxation ... More and more ... Nothing can distract you ... Now, concentrate on your legs ... Feel the way they grow numb ... More and more ... Now, your legs are heavy ... As heavy as lead ... Feel your arms become heavy ... More and more ... Your eyelids grow heavy ... More and more ... Your eyes are hermetically closed ... Now, you can no longer open them ...You no longer want to ... You are sinking gently into this wonderful feeling of fatigue and heaviness ... More and more deeply".

Observe a minute of silence, then resume the suggestions:

"Feel it. A beneficial peace envelops you ... In this state, each of your cells renews itself ... You are quite well ... Soon, I will count to three ... On three, your arms will be light ... You will be able to move them ... You will open your eyes and feel fresh and alert ... One ... Two ... Three ... Open your eyes".

CONTROL QUESTION

Now, question the patient on his reactions. You may receive the following replies.

"I clearly felt relaxation at the following suggestions: 'at each inhalation, you sink more and more deeply into a pleasant sensation of peace and relaxation ... Your arms are heavy ...'

"But, I can still not raise them in spite of the contrary command. However, I could easily have opened my eyes."

Retain this useful information so as to succeed with a second hypnosis. It is necessary to repeat the suggestions:

"Your arms and legs are heavy ... You must close your eyes ..."

Do not repeat those which have proved to be ineffective.

CONCENTRATE ON THE EFFECTIVE SUGGESTIONS

Suggestions to induce the second hypnosis:

"Put yourself at ease ... Slacken the muscles of your arms and legs ... Relax ... Breathe slowly, regularly ... At each inhalation, you sink deeply into a pleasant sensation of peace and relaxation ... Breathe slowly, regularly ... Slowly ... Regularly ... You are quite relaxed ... You are feeling quite well ... At each inhalation, let yourself sink into this wonderful feeling of peace and relaxation ... More and more ... Feel it. This feeling is spreading throughout your body ... And now, concentrate on your arms ... Feel it. Your arms are growing heavy ... More and more ... Now, your arms are heavy ... As lead ... You can no longer raise them ... You can no longer move them ... Your two arms remain motionless ... Your eyes are closed ... Remain closed ... Your breathing is slow and regular ... At each inhalation you sink more and more deeply into a pleasant

sensation of peace and relaxation . . . You are more and more tired . . . More and more".

Observe a minute of silence:

"You are still experiencing this wonderful peace . . . Each of my words is rooted in your subconscious . . . You will carry them out . . . I am going to count to three . . . On three, your arms and legs will be movable and light . . . You will open your eyes and you will feel fresh and alert . . . If I put you once more under hypnosis, you will sink at once into this pleasant state of peace and relaxation . . . You will feel a peace, superior to the previous one, envelop you".

SECOND METHOD OF CONTROLLING THE PATIENT

Question the patient:

"Does the phrasing of the suggestions suit you?"

"Is the tempo too slow or too fast?"

Everything seems perfect. Now, you can contemplate a third hypnosis. Condition the patient: implant a code word in his subconscious which will immediately induce every other hypnotic state. Then, initiate the third hypnosis.

THIRD HYPNOSIS

Suggestions:

"Put Yourself at ease. Slacken the muscles of your arms and legs ... Relax ... Breathe slowly, regularly ... At each inhalation, you sink more and more deeply into this pleasant feeling of peace and relaxation ... Breathe slowly, regularly ... You are quite relaxed ... You are feeling quite well ... At each breath, you sink more and more into this pleasant sensation of fatigue and heaviness ... Feel it. This sensation is spreading through your whole body ..."

Observe a silence of thirty seconds.

"Concentrate on your arms ... Feel it. They are getting heavier and heavier ... More and more ... More and more ... Now, your arms are as heavy as lead ...

You can no longer raise them ... You can no longer move them at all ... Your two arms are as heavy as lead, motionless ... Your eyes are closed ...Remain closed ... Breathe slowly, regularly ... At each inhalation, you sink into the pleasant sensation of peace and relaxation ... More and more ... More and more deeply ... You are sinking into this pleasant sensation of heaviness and fatigue ... You are more and more tired ... More and more."

Pause.

"Nothing can distract you ... You hear only my voice ... Feel it. You are sinking deeper and deeper into a state of beneficial peace ... You are sinking into it more and more ... More and more."

CONDITIONING OF THE PATIENT

"Feel it. In this wonderful state of peace an opening is made to your subconscious ... This opening is growing wider ... All my words are registered by your subconscious ... They are taking

*definite root there . . . You will obey. If I
say the word, KI-AI, your eyes will
close . . . You will fall once more into this
state of peace and relaxation . . . More
and more deeply . . . The word KI-AI will
be enough; you will immediately close
your eyes . . . You will sink into this wonderful state of relaxation and peace . . . It
will be an absolute necessity . . . You will
obey."*

Observe a minute of silence.

*"Soon, I am going to count to three . . .
On three, you will open your eyes . . . You
will be re-awakened, fresh and alert.
But, all my words are definitely rooted
in your subconscious . . . You will obey. If
I say, KI-AI, your eyes will close. You
will sink into this pleasant state of peace
and relaxation. It is an absolute
necessity . . . You will obey. One . . .
Two . . . Three . . . Open your eyes. Feel
it. You are fresh and alert. Your arms
and legs are light, movable . . . You are
full of strength and energy."*

In this text, I have given you a standard example of split hypnosis — or hypnosis followed by a conditioning — which will automatically trigger a series of hypnotic states.

HYPNOSIS BY MEANS
OF TELEVISION

AN AMERICAN EXPERIMENT

An American television company set up an interesting experiment. It announced, "An illusionist will attempt to hypnotize you through your television set. If you do not wish to take part in the experiment, we urge you to switch off your sets at X o'clock".

At the appointed time, the hypnotist spoke his suggestions on television. After a few minutes, he concluded with those which are appropriate for cancelling the hypnotic state.

The television company awaited the viewers' reactions.

THE REACTIONS

On the following days, thousands of letters poured in. Their gist: enthusiasm or displeasure. The latter was expressed by those who, certain they would not succumb, fell into a hypnotic state. Under hypnosis, they had not heard the suggestion discontinuing their state. Great anxiety was felt by those with them. But, the following morning, all re-awakened in good health.

How can this phenomenon be explained?

A LATENT TENDENCY

An experiment such as this certainly has its risks; it demonstrates the following facts:

☐ neither a mysterious fluid nor magnetic irradiation induces hypnosis.

☐ in every human being, a latent tendency to be put under hypnosis exists. The difficulty of the task varies according to the personality of the subject.

Patience overcomes even the most skeptical. According to this theory, no human being should exist who is not hypnosensitive.

DEEP HYPNOSIS

20% of the human race are susceptible to being put under deep hypnosis. In this state, their subconscious is entirely subject to the authority of the hypnotist.

Note that, even under deep hypnosis, commands in conflict with fundamental inclinations and with the personality of the hypnotized subject will automatically suspend the hypnotic state.

Once out of this state, the patient undergoes a form of posthypnotic amnesia. That is to say, once awake, he will remember neither his words nor his actions under deep hypnosis.

The art of medicine pays no attention to this fact. This gives you the opportunity to influence the subconscious.

PREMONITION BY HYPNOSIS

One day, I had transferred a person under deep hypnosis into the future.

Suggestion:

"You are twenty-five years old". (The girl was seventeen years of age.)

She related to me the following events:

"At the age of eighteen, I met my future husband. We had an argument, then went our separate ways. Two years after our reconciliation, we became engaged. Four years after our engagement, we were married. My husband is an engineer in a neighboring factory. Last year, a son, Jochen, was born to us. We purchased a building lot in a nearby vil-

lage. We expect to be able to move into our home for Christmas".

A few years later, I met this young woman. *Everything had taken place according to her predictions under deep hypnosis.* I had the notion of becoming a medium. With no result. This phenomenon of premonition or clairvoyance happened only once in my career.

HOW IS DEEP HYPNOSIS INDUCED

Use the normal methods. Deepen the hypnosis with appropriate suggestions. These will be often repeated. The infallible method is split hypnosis.

HYPNOSIS IN THE VOID

DEFINITION

Hypnosis in the void is a very special form of hypnosis. You begin by inducing the hypnotic state with the usual suggestions. Once the patient is put into this state, stop all suggestions.

You will obtain the correction or elimination of a disturbing factor of the vegetative functions.

RELAXATION-HYPNOSIS AND POST-HYPNOTIC SLEEP

Here is how it's done:

Set off a relaxation-hypnosis by the usual suggestions. Suggest a posthypnotic sleep. Stop all suggestions. Leave the patient in this state 30 minutes or several hours.

Begin the operation once more, this time giving the therapeutic suggestions. Keep the patient in this state for several hours. The hypnosis will deepen.

Another form of hypnosis in the void is uninterrupted hypnosis, or continuous sleep. The patient is taken out of this permanent hypnotic state only at meal-times.

The effect obtained: the patient gains self-knowledge. It is a type of dialogue with self where the will to correct oneself will give shape to the desired personality.

Avoid all possible distraction which would come from the environment.

To summarize: put under this form of hypnosis or under one of its derivatives mentioned above, the patient relives the events suppressed in the dungeons of his memory. These are unknown factors which have been the cause of reprehensible behavior. This type of hypnotherapy eliminates these unknown causes of psychic imbalance.

ANIMAL HYPNOSIS

A state analogous to the hypnotic state can occur among animals. This is the stupor of hares and does in front of car headlights, or the reflex of the lethargic posture of the small animal faced with an overwhelming opponent.

This state may be called cataleptic stiffness due to terror.

This reflex of instinctive immobility is, for the animal, the way to escape danger. By simulating death, it supposes that it becomes unimportant to its adversary. This stiffness, this momentary paralysis, is a protective shield against all external aggression.

Try the experiment.

Take a hen. Set it on its back. Keep it in this position by force, for a short space of time. Once the hen becomes calm, gently remove your hands. It will remain in the position in which it was put. More stimulation will be necessary to make it come out of its state of prostration.

ANOTHER EXPERIMENT

I have known of the reaction of this bird since childhood. On vacation in the country at my aunt's home, I made use of this stratagem to play a joke on her. One by one, I caught the hens. I put them in the position described above, then scattered them around on the steps leading to the house. Imagine ten stiff hens, in a comatose sleep, as if dead . . .To the dismay of my poor aunt, who wept for her beloved birds. I had only to clap my hands once . . .and all the hens, "restored to life", flew away!

Editor's Note:You may also draw a straight chalk line on the ground, lay the hen down on the line, in the same direction on its side, and turn its beak to put it on the line for a few moments. Hypnotized by the line, the hen will remain motionless.

THE CLASSIC METHODS:

You may successfully perform this experiment with any animal. Here are the classic methods:

☐ frighten the animal

☐ look it straight in the eye

☐ prevent its freedom of movement

I.P. Pavlov stated: All conditioned reflexes in animals produce different results, depending on the individual reactions of each of them.

The same technique thus has several effects, on which the hypnotist himself also has an influence.

HYPNOSIS AND CHILDREN

ARE THEY SUGGESTIBLE, HYPNOSENSITIVE?

Children are very suggestible. Nevertheless, to be able to hypnotize them, you must take their age and degree of maturity into consideration. As a general rule, a child can be hypnotized from the age of 9. This faculty tapers off during puberty, returns, then stabilizes in adulthood.

Their attention, attracted and distracted by several subjects at once, is an almost insurmountable obstacle. You can, with difficulty, reach the lower threshold of their consciousness. Discover the art and the manner of manipulating them; a beneficial influence will then be possible for you.

Observation: Children pick up the least hesitation, the slightest lack of assurance on the part of the hypnotist. So be sure of yourself.

Unconsciously, your thoughts are outwardly manifested by gestures or by words. A child will not excuse your slightest hesitation, which gravely compromises the achievement of the desired effect. Thus, an assurance, a never-failing firmness, ensures success, even with very small children.

I have succeeded in being able to hypnotize a few children of seven years old and one little girl of four.

WHAT IS THE APPROPRIATE TECHNIQUE? HOW MAY IT BE ADAPTED?

It is important to find a technique adapted to the world of childhood.

If you are dealing with children under the age of ten, start by indirect hypnosis.

Here is the way. I ask the parents to have the child bring his favorite toy to the first session. They will prepare the child in the following manner:

"We are ill. We are going to visit the healer. You will come with us, and bring your toy bear. Teddy is sick. The healer will help him".

HOW DO YOU INITIATE INDIRECT HYPNOSIS?

I talk to the parents for a moment. We pretend to ignore the child. Then, I turn to the stuffed animal and I ask it:

"Are you ill, Teddy? Where does it hurt?"

Spontaneously, the child gives all possible and imaginable information. I address myself once more to the bear:

"I see that you are ill. But I'm going to cure you. Lie down and close your eyes".

The child will put down "Teddy", who cannot close his eyes. I say to the toy animal's owner:

"Look, your bear is so silly, so tiny! How will he know how to lie down without moving or keep his eyes closed for a long time, if you do not show him how?"

With great goodwill, the child will lie down, motionless, with his eyes closed.

I trigger off the hypnosis by referring to the toy:

"Show Teddy how to be still, how to keep his eyes closed for a long time. You know, he's looking at you. Don't move ...

Show him how to breathe slowly, regularly ... Relax your arms and legs ... Feel it. Your arms and legs are quite light ... Keep your eyes closed ... Teddy's watching you. He's doing what you do.

"You are quite calm ... Have nice dreams now, but you can hear me ... Listen well ... You will obey my commands ... If you do not obey, Teddy will not get better ... You want to obey me, because you want your teddy bear to get better".

In most cases, hypnosis is induced.We can then formulate and apply the suggestions for healing or correction of a given illness or a given instance of bad behavior.

AN EXAMPLE TO STIMULATE SCHOOL-WORK

"You are going to school. Teddy is going too ... But, your bear is now going to listen well to his teacher ... And you too. You won't be distracted any more ... You will apply yourself to working well ... If you know the answer, you will

raise your hand . . . The teacher will be pleased . . . You will conscientiously do your homework . . . You won't go out to play before you've done it. Your handwriting is improving . . . You are writing better and better (etc . . .)".

HOW IS THE CHILD CONDITIONED FOR A SECOND HYPNOSIS?

After having given the above suggestions, do not forget to condition the child with a view to a second hypnosis. Tell him:

"Don't forget my commands . . . You will obey me . . . Now listen well, if I stroke your hair, you will close your eyes. You will not move any more. There, I see you have understood. You will obey".

I repeat:

"When I stroke your hair, you will close your eyes. You will sink into a pleasant feeling of peace . . . I will count to three. On three, you will open your eyes . . . Arms and legs, relaxed, light . . . You will feel quite well. One . . . Two . . .

Three . . . Open your eyes! Feel it. You are in terrific shape"

SECOND HYPNOSIS

After a few visits, all you will have to do is stroke the child's hair. His eyes will close. The hypnosis is triggered off. You have created an atmosphere of trust beforehand. For example, in these terms:

"I am pleased to see you again. I am going to stroke your hair, and straightaway your eyes will close. You will feel the same feeling of peace that you had the first time. You will sink deeply into it. I want only for you to be well".

HOW IS HYPNOSIS INDUCED BY STORIES?

If you have to deal with small children, start by telling them stories. For example:

"Today I will tell you a story. Lie down; close your eyes and listen. Once upon a time, there was a little girl who did not like to go to school. And she never did her homework. Her only desire was to play. Her parents were very distressed

about it. They would have liked so much for their girl to be intelligent and responsible.

"One day, this girl met a very intelligent old man. She told him, 'I don't like school. I just won't go there.'

"And the old gentleman told her, 'Of course, you don't want to go to school now. But you will regret it later. Everything your friends learn will be very useful to you in life. If you are ignorant, you won't find a job. You will never have money, nothing to eat, no toys. But it is never too late to do well. From now on, you will go to school. Go there willingly. Apply yourself. Learn your lessons and do your homework. All the nice things that you want so much, you will be able to buy them.

" 'And, one day, a handsome and intelligent young man will come and marry you. He will be very proud that his girl is so educated! Do you understand why you must go to school? Yes, of course! Now, you will go; you will like learning.'

"And here is the end of my story. This little girl I told you about, worked hard. She became an accomplished and happy young lady. And because you want to become very happy, from now on you will do as the little girl in my story has done".

Note: *Children are excellent collaborators — IF you do not leave the world of childhood.*

SPECIAL CASES: HYPNOSIS AND THE ELDERLY, HYPNOSIS OF DIFFICULT PEOPLE

THE REQUIRED BASIC SUGGESTIONS:

As they grow old, people become less and less hypnosensitive. To induce hypnosis with them, I will give you my procedure. Say:

> *"We will make a test. I would like to know if you can hypnotize yourself. Close your eyes. Hold your arm straight out".*

Now I give the basic suggestions:

> *"Feel it. Your arms are getting heavier and heavier . . . You can hardly hold them straight out . . . This heaviness takes over your arms . . . You can no longer raise them . . . Your arms are beginning to droop . . . More and more . . . Now, they have fallen to your knees".*

If the patient's arms have fallen, give the command:

> *"Open your eyes!"*

No person of that age can keep the arms in that position for more than ten minutes. They will fall automatically. The person will be suggestible in proportion to the rate at which he lowers his arms. Now that he is well conditioned, he will fall easily into a hypnotic state.

ANOTHER EXAMPLE OF A TEST

The patient is seated on a couch or a bed, his legs stretched out, his eyes closed. No elderly person can maintain this position for long.

Suggest:

"Feel it. You are falling backwards ... You are pushed backwards ... More and more ... Now you can no longer keep yourself in a seated position ..."

Any person will naturally tend to return to a more comfortable position. Encourage this tendency by exerting a slight push against the patient's hands. He will have fallen by the time the thirty seconds have passed.

Next, you follow with the basic suggestions.

PEACE, WARMTH AND SECURITY

"Feel it. A wonderful feeling of peace spreads through your whole body . . . Your entire body is enveloped by this feeling of calm and relaxation . . . You are feeling quite well . . . You are sinking deeper and deeper into this wonderful feeling of peace and relaxation . . . You are calm . . . Tired . . . More and more tired.

"Now, I am putting my hand on your stomach . . . Feel it. A beneficial warmth emanates from it . . . This is enveloping you . . . Your muscles are relaxing . . . Loosening . . . You feel quite well . . . Secure . . . I want your well-being . . . I want to help you . . . You are in good hands . . . Give yourself up to this feeling of security."

CONQUERING DISTRESS

Do you have to deal with an individual who is difficult to hypnotize?

In this case, proceed by stages. First, an atmosphere of mutual trust will encourage physical and psychic relaxation, and ease hypnosis. Then eliminate the enemy of relaxation which is *the distress of the patient*. Here is how you do it:

Chat with the subject to be hypnotized. Try to discern the cause of possible distress, to create an atmosphere of security. Never yet give a command. Urge the patient towards a close collaboration. Say, for instance,

"We are going to try to establish a perfect hypnotic rapport. Without your collaboration, we will obtain no result".

HOW DO YOU MAKE YOUR PATIENT DREAM?

Here is the technique.

The patient lies or sits, relaxed, eyes closed. He begins to daydream. Let him describe all the images or impressions perceived.

Guide this dream.

Examples:

1. The patient imagines himself going off on vacation

2. Sees himself climbing a mountain.

All mental images of whatever event are to be described without omitting any detail.

Now question the patient. Obliged to respond, he will make an effort to concentrate on the mental symbols.

You have, by this method, the means of psychoanalyzing the subject. The mental images dreamed are a faithful reflection of the problems to be resolved.

ANOTHER TECHNIQUE: TRANSFORMING PRETENDING TO HYPNOTIC REALITY

The patient feels no result from the hypnosis. But, perhaps to please you, he pretends to do so. In this case, I tell him:

"Feel it. Your eyes are heavy, heavier and heavier ... They are closing".

The patient will slowly close his eyes. But you can see that he is continuing to pretend.

Next, I suggest:

"Feel it. Your eyes want to close ... Try to open them ... You can no longer do it ... Now, you can no longer open your eyes".

The patient will appear to make a superhuman effort to open his eyes. He is still playing the game.

Repeat the procedure several times, one right after the other. As the repetition grows tedious, the patient will end up being caught at his own game. The pretence will become reality.

I will give you an example:

During the last war, many soldiers pretended to have an illness that was apparently serious and incurable, with the intention of being discharged. Once the discharge was obtained, they returned home.

However, some of them continued to fake the symptoms of this supposed illness, so they would not be caught in their deception. As time went on, they suffered the actual, physical symptoms of this imaginary illness.

What had happened? The repetition of the symptoms eventually convinced their subconscious that they in fact did suffer from the disease they had previously only pretended to have.

How can you use this trait? By insisting that your patients tape the actions you want them to manifest after your hypnosis. And then listen to the tapes over and over again, without cease. Soon their subconscious, too, will give way to this repetitive persuasion.

HYPERVENTILATION

"Hyperventilation," or accelerated breathing, is an excellent means of inducing hypnosis.

Tell the patient — who is in a chair — to breathe faster — faster — faster. The patient will breathe in this manner until he feels a slight dizziness.

He will stop, then — under your suggestion — will resume the accelerated respiratory movement. Another dizzy spell will be experienced. Make use of this to trigger off the hypnosis.

Suggest:

"Feel it. Your eyes are becoming heavier and heavier ... Soon your eyes will close".

When the patient has closed his eyes, add:

"During the second session, your eyes will close more quickly".

Perform several sessions of this type. Then his eyes will automatically close after a few seconds.

We have seen that these methods encourage hypnosis and eliminate possible distress. To begin changing the patient, proceed in the same manner as for hypnotizing difficult persons. This, of course, encourages and strengthens the desired effect.

Then, once the patient is out of his hypnotic sleep, question him about his impressions under hypnosis.

Examples:

"Were your arms and legs as heavy as lead?"

"Was it unpleasant?"

"Did you hear me speaking?"

OTHER METHODS

Here is an excellent preparation for hypnosis.

The patient listens to music recorded on cassettes. He rests and relaxes. This very effective method is indispensable for patients enslaved to the stress of modern life. Try it, you will discover its soothing effect.

HOW TO MASSAGE THE REFLEXIVE ZONE OF THE SOLES OF THE FEET

You can strengthen the soothing effect previously obtained by massaging the reflexive zone of the soles of the feet.

Here is how it's done:

This zone is situated slightly below the middle toe, in the center of the sole. Place your thumb on this center.

Carry out the massage by successive pressures, each one lighter than the last. These will be executed simultaneously on both feet.

Then make circles, going from the central point to the edge of the soles. The thumb remains on the reflex point during the execution of the movement. The patient will eventually fall asleep.

LIGHTNING HYPNOSIS AND DIFFICULT PEOPLE

To conclude: All these techniques will allow you to overcome the resistance of the most difficult subjects to hypnotize.

It should be mentioned that, once out of the hypnotic state, the patient should be questioned on the impressions received under hypnosis. The information will be valuable for performing a second hypnosis.

THE CODE WORD

If you intend to hypnotize a patient several times in succession, use hypnosis by code word. This word will be chosen from outside of common speech so as to avoid an accidental hypnosis by posthypnotic command.

Agree upon a word with the patient. Spoken by someone other than yourself, this word should have no effect.

Here is an interesting experiment with a group of patients. A code word must be agreed with each of them
which will set off hypnosis in each participant at the
same moment.

I remember having one day used a code word to put
an entire class under hypnosis. The teacher was overcome
with amazement!

HYPNODIAGNOSIS AND THE ILL

HOW DO YOU TRAIN THE MEMORY?

Under hypnosis, one has an extraordinary memory at one's disposal. Insignificant details, long forgotten, crowd back.

Example: You can obtain the exact description of each object contained in the school satchel of a patient's first beginning of term.

A light hypnosis will suffice to get a detailed recital, impossible in the waking state.

By this means, the sick person will indicate to you the cause of his illness. Its origin is now suppressed in his subconscious by conscious inhibitions, which are obstacles to his recovery.

Put him in hypnosis. When he is there, take him back, ten years at a time, to the moment the illness first occurred, then bring him back to the present without its symptoms.

HOW DO YOU SUGGEST A DREAM?

If the replies to direct questioning do not satisfy you, *make the suggestion of a dream*. This will release details unknown to the conscious mind. The amount of detail is in direct relation to the disturbing factor.

Suggest:

"Your dream will be of short duration. You will reawaken in great form. You will remember everything in detail".

Certain people believe that they cannot dream upon command. In this case, the proposed technique proves effective.

Once the patient is under deep hypnosis, suggest:

"You are quite calm . . . You are under deep hypnosis . . . Very deep . . . You can talk to me . . . You answer my questions . . . With each word spoken, your hypnosis will deepen . . . You will have no difficulty in speaking to me . . . With each word, you will sink into a pleasant feeling of peace and relaxation . . . More and more . . . Your psychic eye clearly perceives the detail responsible for your illness . . . It all comes back into your memory . . . You are reliving the events. Describe what you see in detail . . . Observe what you are experiencing with attention".

THE TRANSPARENT BODY

Under deep hypnosis, you can lead the patient to re-live the traumatic events, question by question. Once the cause of the illness is discovered, you will be able to elim-inate its effects and achieve the cure.

A variation is the following suggestion:

"See, your body is transparent . . . You are in front of a mirror . . . See your or-gans . . . Watch the beating of your heart, the respiratory movement of your lungs. Recognize your vesicle . . . Check it. Is there a stone?"

Such a physical exploration of the body is, of course, impossible. (This classic phenomenon, sometimes sponta-neous, is called "autoscopy.") But your suggestions call on the subconscious to carry out an attentive internal inves-tigation. It is the one sure way of detecting the cause of the illness.

WRITING UNDER HYPNOSIS

Ask the patient to write out, in detail, on paper, the impressions received under hypnosis.

Suggest:

*"With each word written, your hypnosis
will deepen".*

When he comes out of the hypnosis, the surprised
patient does not recognize himself as the author of these
written words. To persuade him, you must compare them
with other writings in his hand.

WHY RECORD ON A TAPE RECORDER?

However, the written description of mental images
leaves out valuable details. Personally, I record all oral
questions and answers on a tape recorder. The wave of
images received will not be stopped by the effort made to
write. This spoken stream of symbols induces a succession
of precise events.

A CASE IN POINT

I recorded the following case:

One day, I received a young woman in my office. I di-
agnosed a constant pain in her lower jaw, an acute neuralgia. The patient, nervously exhausted, was unable to
react positively.

Before undertaking the hypnotherapy, I put her under hypnosis several times to ease the pain. I tried to di-

rect her towards its cause. I questioned her. She answered spontaneously:

"Three years ago, my husband and I were on vacation. He was unfaithful to me with a seasonal waitress staying on the same floor. Six months later, I learned of my misfortune. I wanted a divorce. But my husband swore that he would never again yield to this type of adventure, since it was also painful for him.

"I no longer ate. I no longer slept. I grew visibly thinner. A treatment caused me to regain my appetite. I began to eat continuously. I gained 10 pounds in no time at all!

"Since then, this pain in the lower jaw began. At first, every two or three days; then, night and day".

I made the following deduction: hate towards her rival manifested itself as neuralgia. My advice was for her to invite this woman and have it out with her over a cup of coffee, then forget the adventure.

The patient, shocked, refused to do it. I abandoned the case. But my patient came to consult with me a few days later. She promised to follow my advice. She implored me to continue the hypnotic treatment, which I did.

She was certainly cured, for I never heard her speak of this woman again.

MEANS AND LIMITS OF HYPNOSIS

SURPRISING PHENOMENA

HOW DO YOU STIMULATE VITALITY?

HOW DO YOU SHARPEN THE SENSES?

The capabilities of the neuro-vegetative system are immeasurable. They come into play under hypnosis.

Examples:

☐ In the hypnotic state, *muscular strength is clearly superior to that shown in the waking state.*

☐ Under hypnosis, *perfect relaxation is achieved.* It is impossible to attain this in the waking state. The conscious mind is an obstacle to relaxation.

☐ In hypnosis, you hold the means of *influencing inner functions. For example, you can accelerate or slow down the rate of heartbeat.*

HERE IS AN EXPERIMENT

To what extent can one sharpen the senses?

The following experiment will give you the answer.

Take a new pack of cards which are all identical to the touch. Choose one of them. Note its color and value. Put someone under deep hypnosis.

Command:

"Open your eyes!"

Show him the back of the selected card. Suggest:

"I will show you this card a second time. You will notice a black cross on its back. You will recognize the card by this sign".

Put the card in question back into the pack. Shuffle. Show the back of each one in turn to the person undergoing the experiment.

Say:

"Recognize the card marked with a distinctive sign".

As a general rule, the hypnotized subject will point it out, in spite of the absence of the cross.

PRODUCING A BLISTER BY MEANS OF SUGGESTION

A committee of doctors observed an experiment, the result of which was drawn up in a report. It concerned the development of a blister, due to a suggestion of a burn.

This is what happened.

The hypnotist touched the person's skin with a cold metallic object, a coin. He suggested:

"Feel it. The coin is very hot. It is burning your skin".

This suggestion given, the patient was awakened. All present noticed the formation of a blister at the place where the object was applied.

OTHER EXAMPLES

Platonov relates in his book, *Das Wort als Physiologischer und Heilender Faktor*:

N.I. Finne put a person thirty-eight years of age under hypnosis. He placed a copper coin on the inner side of his forearm.

Suggestion:

> *"We have just put a burning coin on your arm. You will receive a painful burn".*

This suggestion was repeated several times. One of the physicians observed the subject very closely once he was out of the hypnotic state. Here is his report:

"Twenty-five minutes after the awakening of the subject undergoing the experiment, a diffuse redness appeared at the place touched by the coin. After fifty-five minutes, the spot was swollen. After an hour and a half, a white spot was seen at the center of the burn. At the end of three hours and thirty minutes, a blister typical of burns took shape".

What process produced this phenomenon? No valid explanation has been put forward on this subject. Schaefer comments:

"In attempting to explain this suggestive burn, followed by the formation of a blister, let us not forget the following factor. This phenomenon occurs without any physical intervention (scratching of the skin), by the patient. Consequently, it is the result of a nervous impulse. But such an explanation appears debatable for two definite reasons.

How can a simple excitation of sympathetic nerves, leading to the epidermis, create a blister? We know that the latter is the effect of a local destruction of cells and of a lesion of blood vessels, caused by the agency of a high temperature.

We also note that the nervous system sustains the same intensity of excitation throughout. But the arm has only one blister!

In conclusion: "The impulses responsible for a single suggestive blister in a given spot as yet escapes our comprehension".

(Quotation from: V. Safonov, *Wissenschaft und Religion*, 1967).

WALKING ON FIRE, A PUZZLING PHENOMENON

In his journal, *Deutschen Medizinischen Wochenschrift*, no. 32. 1940, B. Buschan relates:

"The first descriptions of this phenomenon were brought to our attention by Saporta who observed it in Polynesia, on the island Raya-Taja.

"A priest walked on burning stones while praying, without receiving the slightest burn. The spectators, previously conditioned, mentally supported him. The condition given by the priest, 'The world will ignite in a tremendous blaze if one of the participants at the ceremony withdraws in fear' ".

Kellogg observed this phenomenon in Tahiti:

"Stones were heated for two days and two nights. Then natives walked on this burning path, twelve yards long. I tried to draw close to it. The great heat given off by it made me retreat several yards. I threw an old shoe at it, and it burned up in the wink of an eye. The feet of the walkers bore no trace of a wound".

Wirtz attended this type of ceremony in India:

"The pilgrims walked towards the images of their gods, barefoot, on burning coals. Their objective was to decorate them with flowers and garlands. None of them suffered the slightest burn".

Johnson attended this type of ceremony in Martinique:

"They walk along a path, seven yards in length, made of burning coals. The heat coming from it radiates to a distance of ten yards. On each side of this blaze are images of their gods. The reason for the ceremony is to bring sacrificial offerings.

"The high priest, talismans in hand, heads the procession. His gaze, unmoving, is fixed on the idols. He appears to be unaware of the heat of the fire. His feet sink into it up to the ankles. All at once, his face loses its stiffness. But he goes on to the end!

"The following priest wears flowers on his head. His steps are steady and sure. Suddenly, half way along, his strength seems to desert him . . . He is going to fall! . . . No . . . A reserve of energy carries him to the end!

"Three men and three women are next. Novices. Their posture is mouth open, glassy look, lost is a fog. All at once, one of the women begins to scream. The priest strikes her on the head with a wet rope. With an uncertain step, she drags herself to the other end of the fire.

"Absolutely all the participants had their feet free of any burn!"

Cowell reports from Japan:

"This ceremony takes place twice a year in a little temple in Ontaka. Burning coals are laid on a path four yards long and one yard wide. On each side are sacred texts. The fire is fanned by broad swinging panels attached to long sticks.

"A group of priests heads the procession. From the latter, a congregation separates, led by the high priest who walks with a confident step over the fire".

A CONTROLLED EXPERIMENT

In 1935, the members of an association of researchers on the subject prepared a report of such an experiment, carried out by fakir Kuda Baks. (H. Price, University of London, Council for Psychological Investigations). Here is an excerpt from this report.

"Before initiating the experiment, the fakir's feet were carefully washed and examined. No trace of any possible preparation. The soles of the feet were soft and dry! The temperature of the skin was 86 degrees.

"Two furnaces, one ten feet long, the other four feet wide, were filled with newspapers, paraffin and kindling. Over these materials, a layer of coal was spread. The fire was lit at Eight A.M. At Four P.M., the time of the ceremony, the furnaces were incandescent blazes. The whole experiment was photographed and filmed. Without haste, the fakir went back and forth, in five steps, on the first furnace. The temperature of the epidermis was 86 degrees. The soles of the feet were unharmed. He got ready to cross the second furnace. Suddenly, he turned toward the inspection committee, visibly annoyed:

" 'Something has distracted and thwarted me. I have lost control of myself. I cannot resume the experiment'.

"A member of this committee attempted to carry out the experiment. After two steps, he fled screaming with pain! His feet, badly burned, were under treatment in the hospital for a long time!

"I wished to be an eyewitness to such an event."

EVENTS EXPERIENCED

I extended an invitation to an Indian yogi. He was my guest for a few weeks, enough time to study and photograph the various experiments.

First experiment:

We buried the yogi for two hours in a plastic bag. He came out of it unhurt. Not the slightest lesion was in evidence!

Second experiment:

His eyes blindfolded, he used a bow and arrows to shoot at seven threads, from which weights were suspended. He severed the seven threads simultaneously!

Third experiment:

I lit a pile of beech wood. After four hours, an unbearable heat was being given off by it. The yogi, Ram Preja Dass, went around the fire while praying. Then, he crossed the blaze three times. I remained as though petrified! Pulling myself together, I ran to his aid. A useless gesture: his feet were perfectly unharmed!

HOW DO YOU COMBAT PAIN?

Hypnosis, the hypnosis of others and self-hypnosis, exert their beneficial effect in many fields. *Above all, they relieve pain.* Many painful surgical operations have been performed under hypnotic anaesthesia. Detailed descriptions of this type of operation no longer allow the effectiveness of hypnosis to remain in doubt.

Consequently, any pain, no matter how great, can be neutralized under hypnosis. Above all, imaginary pain such as certain headaches, are often eliminated by hypnotherapy.

THE OBJECTIVE LIMIT

FLIGHT INTO ILLNESS

The ways of healing offered by hypnosis are nonetheless limited.

Example:

If a patient, ill-at-ease, takes refuge in illness, hypnotherapy will come up time and again against the impenetrable screen of self-defense.

Almost all our headaches are the fruits or the symptomatic effects of our problems. The only effective way to contend with them is for us to modify our negative point of view ourselves.

DESIRE, AN OBSTACLE TO SUCCESS

This is the rule to be observed:

Hypnotherapy will be beneficial if no desire opposed to its motivation prevents it from being effected.

If one abides by this law, it will not be restricted only to psychic illnesses.

A simple wound will heal more quickly with hypnotic suggestion.

Any convalescent will recover more rapidly from a successful operation, thanks to positive suggestions.

Here is a phenomenon known to physicians:

A sick person, unhappy in his private or professional life, and made to feel secure by the solicitude of the hospital staff, will heal less quickly than his neighbor who is driven by the desire to leave the hospital as soon as possible.

Volume IV

Master Secrets of Self-Hypnosis

EDITOR'S PREFACE

This final volume of the *Secret Techniques of Hypnosis* is doubtless the one that will be the most useful to you as an individual.

Through self-hypnosis, you will get rid of insomnia and stress.

You will become younger and more beautiful.

You will improve your athletic performance.

And your love life and your sex life will get infinitely better.

Through all these examples, you will be shown the exact words to use . . . to establish immediate, positive suggestions that work.

This system, somewhat like an old wizard's book of magic, is full of formulas which allow you to create amazing phenomena.

However, we want you to gradually become capable of creating these suggestions yourself, enriching them, making them complete, and transposing them — not only to yourself — but to each new case which presents itself to you.

You will see a judicious selection of these formulas that, when they were recorded on cassettes, have often totally transformed the lives of men and women who needed help. What would have become of them if they had not met a hypnotherapist? Their lives would doubtless have been wasted forevermore.

Prof. Tepperwein quotes relatively few examples in the field of health . . . he no doubt wants to avoid any problem with the Medical Association.

However, if you read between the lines, you will be able to discern the extraordinary tool that self-hypnosis can represent to cure any psychosomatic illness.

If you can cure a migraine that has been stubborn for years, expand one breast and then the other in a flat-chested young woman — all with the aid of simple suggestions — then imagine the feats you may achieve over asthma, hay fever, gastric ulcers, and — why not? — more serious illnesses!

You will also be able to give significant help to those who are in pain, thanks again to the techniques of hypnosis.

Of course, if you are not a physician, this field will be barred to you. You will, however, be able to sustain the morale of the sick, who are attended by their doctors, and give them back their smile. And when a patient's morale is skyrocketed, one may expect spectacular cures.

Yes, through self-hypnosis, you will direct the Grand Master of your emotions, your success and your health . . . your subconscious.

YOU NOW HOLD IN YOUR HANDS ONE OF THE GREAT KEYS TO HEALTH AND HAPPINESS: SELF-HYPNOSIS

What is more, as the works of N. Hill and of Murphy show us, self-hypnosis is also one of the keys to riches and abundance.

You now have then means to do it. From this point on, your success depends only on the devotion you give to its principles.

With all my wishes for Health, Happiness and Success . . . thanks to self-hypnosis.

Hypnotically yours,

Christian H. Godefroy,

Editor

SELF-HYPNOSIS:
A WAY TO HELP YOURSELF

HOW PROBLEMS CREATE ILLNESSES

Poor psychic behavior creates physical disturbances. Here is the procedure:

Unresolved problems take root in your subconscious. Disorders result, then illness.

It is no exaggeration if I allow myself to state:

Problems create illness. Heart ailments, neuralgia of the stomach, the head and the back, muscular contractions, insomnia despite fatigue, the feeling of being exhausted, are symptoms exhibited daily to the doctor.

If the results of laboratory analyses of the above maladies are reassuring, the practitioner will conclude:

Your organs are healthy. Your discomfort is due to functional disorders.

Here are the causes: bad habits, occupational demands, stress and nervousness.

These are magnified by lack of exercise, and re-
pressed and unresolved difficulties which are transformed
to weak organs.

The illness then breaks out, and creates new problems . . . The vicious circle is established.

The physician will feel unequal to the task and will
tell you:

"I will prescribe something that will give you relief".

But he knows for a fact that this remedy will eliminate the symptoms and not the cause.

HOW DO YOU HELP YOURSELF THROUGH THE MIND?

In such a case, one solution forces itself on us: healing through the mind.

We know this: any thought that is motivated by a
feeling tends to become reality.

Nevertheless, not everything that we imagine in
thought necessarily becomes reality. Certain indispensable conditions, such as desire and its motivation, give it
an enormous creative force.

Let me quote an example taken from the book by A.
J. Efremor — *Auf Messers Schneide.*

WARMING YOURSELF THROUGH SUGGESTION

"A glacial wind pierced Dayaram like a knife . . . Suddenly, he stopped, stupefied . . . On a rocky projection, stood four naked men. Splashed by the waves, covered with snow, they remained there, motionless. They appeared to be statues carved from yellow stone. But their breath, carried by the wind, proved them to be alive. One of them bent over, soaked a piece of cloth in the water, then used it to cover his back exposed to the glacial wind . . .

"Dayaram remembered having looked at photographs of naked lamas, standing in snowbanks on Mount Kailas. According to a Tibetan theory of mysticism, people like this draw from the very essence of their being an energy called 'Tumo'. This spreads its warmth throughout the body by innumerable channels. Novices, chosen with care, prepare themselves, in successive stages, for such exercises. Clad in light cotton clothing, they begin by breathing in the cold air. Little by little, they get rid of their clothes.

"Special exercises earn them the title 'Respa'. The candidates sit on the ground on the bank of a river or the shore of a lake. They soak pieces of cloth in the water, then wrap themselves in them. The warmth of their bodies should dry them. Formerly, a Respa had to dry three pieces of cloth. He is able to withstand glacial cold for twelve to twenty-four hours.

"The warmth of clothing is replaced by a suggestive fire. Some ascetics, clad in a light cotton loincloth, spend the winter in caves within snowy mountains.

"Under self-hypnosis, the Respa gives himself suggestions which produce an impression of internal fire, or else they imagine a valley burnt by the sun."

AN ENORMOUS POWER

The following example will prove to you the immeasurable power of self-hypnosis. Sven Hedins was travelling across Tibet. One of his colleagues got into an argument with a Tibetan hermit. The latter predicted:

"Next year, on this very day, you will die".

Doctor H., convinced of the extraordinary gifts of Tibetans, believed in this prophecy.

One year later, shortly before the given day, he returned to Berlin. Ill, he put himself in the care of dismayed physicians. All treatment proved ineffective. He was hospitalized. But he wasted away day by day.

The prophecy was therefore mentioned to the chief physician. He immediately ascribed the illness to a destructive self-hypnosis.

He put the patient under hypnosis for four days. Two days after the fatal day, he awakened him and assured him, "Nothing happened. You are still alive".

The suggestion was thus erased and the sick man healed quickly.

Under self-hypnosis, you may use the power of suggestion in a positive way. It is the only means of fulfilling your desires.

STOPPING SMOKING WITH THE HELP OF SELF-HYPNOSIS

I will now explain infallible procedures:

One out of two smokers would like to stop smoking. Often, he has already tried to do so, in vain. Some have held out for a few months, then have relapsed.

HOW CAN ONE RESIST?

Such was the case of Mr. Wagner. This man had succeeded in life. His ideas as the chief executive officer of an insurance company of some substance were effective and obeyed. On the twenty-fifth anniversary of the execution of his duties, mention was made of his iron will and his exemplary discipline.

But in spite of his good qualities, he had not been able to stop smoking. His state of health demanded it. Several attempts met with no result. He had confided his intention to give up cigarettes to his friends.

A new attempt, a new failure! His friends made fun of him. He lost all confidence in himself. In despair, he came to me for a consultation. I reassured him as follows:

"Last year, I treated thousands of smokers. Not one has relapsed. Your problem will be resolved by acupuncture".

This solution did not interest him. He was looking for a way which would allow him to overcome his mania by himself and recover his confidence.

OVERCOMING A BAD HABIT BY MEANS OF A CASSETTE

In this situation, self-hypnosis was indicated. I urged him to record the following on magnetic tape:

"I am lying down, eyes closed, relaxed ... My arms and legs are flexible ... I am quite relaxed ... Nothing can distract me ... I am quite calm ... I let myself be drawn along. I am breathing slowly, regularly ... I am feeling

quite well ... A pleasant peacefulness envelops my body".

At this point, the patient observes a minute of silence.

"Now, I am concentrating on my legs ... I am quite calm ... I clearly feel them growing heavy ... More and more ... Now, my legs are quite heavy. As heavy as lead.

"My arms are growing heavy ... They are drawn downward ... This heaviness pervades my arms more and more ... More and more ... Now, my arms are as heavy as lead.

"My eyelids are heavy ... Heavier and heavier ... My eyes are hermetically closed ... I can no longer open them ... I no longer want to ... I let myself sink more and more into this wonderful feeling of tiredness and heaviness ... I am more and more tired ... More and more tired."

At this stage, the patient observes a minute of silence.

"Nothing can distract me . . . I hear only my voice . . . I feel myself sinking still more, more and more deeply into this feeling of peace . . . I feel quite well . . . I am sinking deeper and deeper . . . More and more."

HOW IS THE SUBCONSCIOUS ADDRESSED?

"In this wonderful state of peace, I have an opening to my subconscious . . . I am learning to resist cigarettes . . . I no longer want to smoke . . . I have no interest in it anymore . . . Smoking no longer interests me at all . . . The very idea is repugnant to me . . . Every time I breathe smoke, I experience this repugnance . . .

"Now, I will not smoke any more . . . Nothing can make me change my mind . . . I am happy to be able to improve my state of health by stopping smoking . . . Day by day, my health is improving . . . I will not smoke any more."

HOW IS REPUGNANCE FOR CIGARETTES SUGGESTED?

"Day by day, I am better at resisting my desire to smoke . . . I no longer experience any interest in smoking . . . The very idea is enough to cause a repugnance for cigarettes. . . . As soon as I breathe smoke, my repugnance increases . . . I am very happy not to smoke any more . . . Nothing can make me change my mind . . . I will never smoke again."

At this point, the patient observes a minute of silence.

Mr. Wagner had promised to listen to this cassette at least once a day. Full of hope, he left my office. I heard nothing more, but months later I received a case of champagne, accompanied by a card. I read there the single word — "Thanks".

Use this method to quit smoking yourself. It is not complicated to put yourself into a hypnotic state sufficent to do this. Simply lie down, or seat yourself in a calm and comfortable place. Close your eyes. Then, listen to a cassette. Here is what you will have recorded:

"I am quite calm . . . Relaxed . . . My arms and legs are flexible . . . A wonder-

*ful peacefulness envelops me . . . My
arms and legs are becoming heavier and
heavier . . . Heavier and heavier . . . I am
sinking deeper and deeper into this
wonderful feeling of tiredness and heaviness . . . I am more and more tired . . .
More and more tired".*

You will repeat these suggestions until this feeling of peace is achieved. No stray thought will make you deviate from your objective.

Remember, too, that other faults can be corrected under self-hypnosis.

HOW IS SELF-HYPNOSIS TESTED?

Before telling you about the usefulness of self-hypnosis, I will describe for you a test that is simple to do. This is the "test of anesthesia". It will give you a precise and concrete notion of the degree of effectiveness of your suggestion.

For example, tell yourself:

"All sensation is disappearing from my left arm".

Repeat this suggestion several times. Next, pinch your arm forcefully to determine to what extent it is free of pain.

As it becomes more and more numb, you will become more and more confident of your control over your unconscious.

EXTRA BONUS

HOW TO NUMB COMPLETELY THE TASTE BUDS THAT DRIVE YOU TO SMOKE, AND NOT EAT AN EXTRA MORSEL TO MAKE UP FOR IT.

Following the commands I gave you above, simply add these to your tape:

"I am opening my body to my mind . . . I can now feel my mind touch and command the inside of my body . . . I am concentrating on my tongue . . . My tongue is now completely under the control of my mind . . . From this moment on, my tongue will numb itself to the taste of cigarettes . . . Every time I light up a cigarette, I will be unable to taste it . . . There will be no pleasure in it . . . There will be no kick in it . . . It will feel dead in my mouth . . . Only a harsh, ugly, burning piece of paper in my mouth".

"And now I go on to command my body to not miss those cigarettes in the slight-

est . . . Since they are so repugnant, since they no longer give me any taste thrill at all, I need put nothing else into my mouth to make up for them . . . I am thrilled to be free of them . . . I need no extra food to make up for them . . . I will not eat one extra morsel to make up for those disgusting cigarettes . . . Not one extra sweet . . . Not one extra piece of candy or cake . . . Not one extra snack . . . I am free . . . I am healthy . . . I am satisfied.

"I feel a wonderful peace coming over me . . . In this state, each one of my words takes root in my subconscious . . . I will behave according to these commands . . . I feel quite well in my position . . . Day by day, my condition improves . . .

"I will soon count up to three . . . On three, my arms and legs will be flexible, moveable once more . . . I will open my eyes . . . I will feel fresh and alert . . . One . . . Two . . . Three . . . I am opening my eyes! My arms and legs are flexible

and moveable ... I am full of strength and energy ... I am feeling quite well".

LOSING STARTLING AMOUNTS OF WEIGHT WITH SELF-HYPNOSIS

This method is particularly suitable for undertaking a weight loss cure. Over 70% of Americans suffer from an overweight condition.

WHAT ARE THE PROBLEMS DUE TO OBE-SITY?

Mrs. Berger had a weight problem. She came to consult me. She had followed a number of diets. No result! Since then, she sought desperately to control her voracious appetite.

When she got married, eight years before, she was young, slender, pretty and lively. After the birth of her daughter, Sabina, she recovered her waspwaist. The attentions showered on her daughter kept her busy ... Then they became routine ...

Boredom took hold. She tried to relieve it by occasional nibbling at candy. This became the object of her gluttony. Her husband saw his wife gain fifteen pounds in a short time. He asked for a divorce, insensitive to his wife's problems.

Anxious to get him back, Mrs. Berger came to consult me. I showed her how to put herself into a hypnotic state. I urged her to record the following suggestions on tape.

SUGGESTIONS REQUIRED FOR OVERCOMING GLUTTONY

"I feel it, candy repels me . . . Day by day, this repugnance increases . . . From this moment, I will eat no more of it . . . I lose pounds each week . . . I feel considerably better . . . I have lost my voracious appetite . . . I take two meals a day . . . I no longer eat snacks . . . As long as I keep listening to this cassette, I will lose pounds per week . . . Day by day, my health improves . . . My digestion works marvelously . . . Eating no longer interests me . . . I feel quite well . . . I eat little at each meal . . . I no longer nibble at candy . . . Day by day, sweets repel me more . . . Each week, I lose pounds of weight . . . I feel very well because of it . . . While listening to this cassette, I will be calm, light, each of my words takes root in my subconscious . . . I will

carry out these commands . . . I feel better, day by day."

The following year, I met Mrs. Berger at a reception — transformed, slender, almost unrecognizable. She had just been remarried to her husband. He had noticed the change in his ex-wife during frequent visits to his daughter. He fell in love all over again!

Another woman, a famous French model, lost 30 pounds so easily that she has now kept it off for 15 years.

HOW TO CONVINCE YOUR BODY THAT IT MUST BURN FAT LIKE A TEENAGER

Record the following suggestions on tape, and play them to yourself once a day:

"I am resting, calm, relaxed, my eyes closed. My arms and legs are flexible . . . I feel free, relaxed . . . Nothing distracts me . . . I let myself be drawn along . . . I am breathing slowly, regularly . . . I am quite relaxed . . . A wonderful peacefulness envelops my body.

"In this state of peace, I have an opening to my subconscious . . . This opening grows wider . . . More and more . . . My

words are settling into my subconscious . . . Are taking root there . . . I will carry out these commands.

"I am reaching down into the cells of my body . . . I can feel my mind entering every swollen fat cell of my body . . . I can feel my entire body becoming warmer and warmer, as the heat rises in every cell.

"New youth is pouring into my body . . . New youth is pouring into every cell of my body . . . I can feel the cells of my body moving backward in time . . . Years and years of age are evaporating from the cells of my body . . . The cells are becoming younger and younger . . . the fat-burning power is becoming stronger and stronger.

"I can feel my body regaining the youth and vitality and fat-burning power of a teenager . . . I can feel the fat in my cells being ignited by this new fat-burning power . . . In every one of my cells, fat is being fed into the furnace . . . Fat is being burned into heat and water . . . The

water is moving into my blood stream, ready to be poured out . . . Each cell is shrinking . . . My entire body is shrinking . . . I am burning fat moment by moment . . . my entire body is slimming itself, moment by moment.

"My body is regaining the youth and power it had when it was a teenager . . . The heat from the fat it burns is being converted into boundless new stores of energy . . . I find that I can work harder, play harder, without getting hungry . . . I no longer have the need to gorge myself . . . I no longer have the need to binge . . . I no longer have the need to have more than a piece of bread between meals.

"Fat is pouring out of my new teenage body . . . I am becoming the person I always wanted to be . . . I am happy with myself . . . I am proud of myself".

HOW TO GET RID OF INSOMNIA BY SELF-HYPNOSIS

Cervantes wrote in his work, *Don Quixote*, "God bless the inventor of sleep". Unfortunately, a large number of people no longer benefit from this wonderful "invention". One in seven of us suffers from insomnia. As a result, millions swallow barbiturates. Over the years, the consumption of these remedies has increased 500 percent.

Are you one of these insomniacs? Begin by determining the cause of this evil. If it is of organic origin, put yourself into the care of a physician.

If not, have recourse to a natural method: self-hypnosis.

SUGGESTION

Record the following suggestions on a cassette in a calm, monotonous voice:

"I am resting, calm, relaxed, my eyes closed. My arms and legs are flexible ... I feel free, relaxed ... Nothing distracts me ... I let myself be drawn along ... I am breathing slowly, regularly ... I am quite relaxed ... A wonderful peacefulness envelops my body".

At this point, observe a minute of silence.

*"Now, I am concentrating on my legs . . .
They are growing heavier and heavier
. . . Now, my legs are as heavy as
lead . . . My arms are getting heavy . . .
Are drawn downwards . . . They are
becoming heavier and heavier . . . My
arms are as heavy as lead . . . My eyes
become heavy . . . More and more . . .
More and more . . . My eyes are
hermetically closed . . . I can no longer
open them . . . I no longer want to do
so . . . I am letting myself sink deeply
into this wonderful feeling of tiredness
and heaviness . . . Into this feeling of
peace . . . "*

AN EXCELLENT WAY TO FALL ASLEEP

*"In this state of peace, I have an opening
to my subconscious . . . This opening
grows wider . . . More and more . . . My
words are settling into my subconscious . . . Are taking root there . . . I will
carry out these commands.*

"The peace is profound . . . A wonderful feeling of quietude and harmony spreads through my body . . . I am cheerful and happy . . . Every evening, upon going to bed, this feeling of peace will surround me. I fall asleep immediately . . . My sleep is healthy, natural . . . On awakening, I will be in good form and rested . . . I will feel this peace and harmony envelop me; I will be cheerful and happy . . . Day by day, everything is better and better."

HOW TO TRANSPORT YOURSELF BACK TO THE DEEP SLEEP YOU HAD AS A CHILD

"Each evening, when going to bed, I eliminate all worrisome thoughts . . . I fall asleep at once . . . I sleep all night until morning . . . I go back in this sleep to the happiest nights I had as a child . . . I am loved . . . I am cared for . . . There is nothing to worry about . . . No one can harm me . . . I can sleep deeply, comfortably, knowing that a beautiful world will be waiting for me on the other side of my beautiful dreams.

*"On awakening, this wonderful feeling
of peace and harmony will surround
me . . . I am cheerful and happy . . . Day
by day, my condition improves . . . Now,
I fall into a deep, healthy sleep until
morning . . . I am sleeping deeply . . .
Deeply."*

Listen to this cassette every evening for several
weeks. Day by day, you will sleep better and better. Little
by little, you will be able to do without the suggestions
recorded on tape. Your problem of insomnia will be resolved.

You can resolve different problems in this way. It is
enough to formulate suggestions according to your desire.
These suggestions will be recorded by your subconscious.

HOW TO IMPROVE SCHOOL-WORK BY SELF-HYPNOSIS

AN EXAMPLE

Throughout his school years, Manfred was one of the best in his class. His parents ran a supermarket and scarcely bothered with their son. They thought that it was unnecessary. Manfred did his homework conscientiously.

Imagine the parents' surprise at the news that their son was not to be advanced to the next grade with his friends! Here is the cause of it. He had gotten it into his head to be a forest ranger. But, destined to take over the family business, he no longer felt obliged to work at school. His work had been motivated by this profession, which, however, remained only a dream . . .

Manfred came to the consultation as a complete dunce. I promised his parents to do what I could to cure his willful laziness. The child was enthusiastic at the prospect of undergoing hypnosis. I urged him to lie down on the couch and listen to my words. I forbade him to make any effort. This remained the privilege of the subconscious.

HOW DO YOU INDUCE HYPNOSIS?

I switched on the tape recorder and induced the hypnosis in these terms:

"Settle yourself comfortably . . . Close your eyes. Relax . . . Your arms and legs are flexible . . . Your eyes are hermetically closed . . . You are more and more tired . . . Surrender to this feeling of tiredness . . . You are quite passive . . . You are concentrating on my voice, which is guiding you . . . You are breathing slowly, regularly . . . You are quite relaxed . . . Nothing distracts you. You are listening only to my words . . . You are quite passive . . . Your breathing is slow, regular . . . Feel it. Your arms are becoming numb . . . They are becoming heavier and heavier . . . Heavier and heavier".

At this point, I observe a minute of silence.

"Feel it. You are sinking deeply into this pleasant feeling of tiredness and heaviness . . . You hear only my voice . . . Now, your legs are becoming heavier and heavier . . . You are breathing slowly,

regularly ... You are feeling quite well. You are surrendering more and more to this wonderful feeling of fatigue and heaviness ... You are more and more tired ... More and more tired."

At this stage, I observe another minute of silence.

"You have an opening to your subconscious ... It gets wider and wider in this wonderful state of peace ... All my words are taking root in your subconscious ... You will carry out my commands."

THE SUGGESTION

"From now on you will concentrate on the words of your teacher ... You will not allow yourself to be distracted ... You will raise your hand each time you know the answer to a question ... You will participate enthusiastically in your class ...

"You will do your homework conscientiously. You will concentrate on your lessons. You will not let yourself be dis-

tracted ... You will not undertake anything else before having finished your homework ... You will prepare the following day's lessons ... Your school activity increases ... You are happy with the results. Day by day, you improve your school performance ... You work with pleasure ... Your school work improves day by day ... Day by day, your schoolwork improves."

HOW DO YOU BRING YOURSELF OUT OF THE HYPNOSIS?

I observe a minute of silence, then I bring him out of the hypnosis in these terms:

"Feel it. A wonderful peace envelops you ... In this state, each of my words takes root in your subconscious ... You will carry out my commands ... I will soon count to three ... On three, your arms and legs will be flexible, moveable again ... You will open your eyes and you will be fresh and alert ... One ... Two ... Three ..."

Manfred opened his eyes. I urged him to listen to the cassette at least once a day, or better still, at least two or three times a day. Enthusiastic about hypnosis, he promised me to do it.

Some weeks later, I received a letter from the child. He had passed his examinations. He advanced to the higher class.

Record your suggestions on a cassette if you have children whose school work leaves room for improvement. Spoken in a calm, monotone voice, they will ensure a positive result.

THE PHENOMENON OF AUTOMATIC FLIRTATIOUSNESS

A large part of our behavior is only the intensification of certain habits to which we have been conditioned throughout our life. Can you get rid of them? Only one means — hypnosis — allows you to rebuild an ideal personality according to your desires.

Mrs. Benner, a beautiful, witty woman, had unknowingly acquired a certain habit. The attention of those present invariably centered on her brilliant personality, the cynosure of society. Apart from rare headaches, she was what one may call the personification of perfect happiness.

She married Professor Benner, neurologist emeritus, and tennis champion. At the time of their engagement, the headaches had disappeared. Then they married . . .

As a speaker of rare ability, the presence of her spouse was in great demand, and he was the center of attention at every party, every gathering which he attended, accompanied by his wife.

As soon as a party promised to be interesting because of the fascinating stories of Mr. Benner, his wife withdrew, the victim of unbearable migraine headaches. Once home again, accompanied by her husband, they disappeared as if by enchantment,

AWAKENING POSITIVE FEELINGS

This type of incident became habitual. Mr. Benner soon put forward a diagnosis. For years, beauty and intelligence had placed his spouse in the front rank of society. At present, she felt dethroned, crushed by her husband's personality.

Her headaches robbed her of her last chance to perch at her usual level. The migraines became an automatic manifestation. Frequent quarrels between the two of them resulted. Mrs. Benner began to drown her sorrows in alcohol, then no longer sobered up all day.

Tired of this situation and unable to reason with his wife, who refused all help from him, Mr. Benner telephoned me. He was a very old friend, opposed to hypnosis.

We arranged a dinner during which I tried to persuade Mrs. Benner of the urgency of treatment. This was easy. Apparently, she had already sought a solution to her problem.

She came to me for consultation. I resolved to treat her in stages. With her consent, I began by eliminating her unhealthy flirtatiousness, her basic problem. After several weeks, this was definitely resolved.

Now, only one part of the treatment remained: to restore her self-confidence. Together, we worked out the suggestions to be recorded on cassette.

CURED IN A FEW WEEKS

"I am quite calm ... My muscles are flexible ... My nerves are relaxed ... I am feeling quite well ... Nothing can distract me ... I am breathing slowly, regularly ... With each breath, I sink more and more into a pleasant sensation of fatigue and heaviness ... I am becoming more and more tired ... More and more ... This wonderful sensation of peace and security covers me like a

cloak . . . I surrender to it . . . Nothing is important any more . . . I am letting myself go . . . All my problems are being resolved . . . I feel free . . . Quite well . . . It is wonderful to let myself go . . . I am sinking deeper and deeper into this beneficial peacefulness. Now, I feel quite free, relaxed . . . And I am concentrating on the words that follow.

"I am quite calm . . . Quite calm . . . A wonderful feeling of peace and harmony spreads through my body . . . I am happy and cheerful . . . My circulation is regular and my digestion is excellent. At any time, I can relax . . . My head remains cool . . . My head is light . . . The nape of my neck and my shoulders are flexible and relaxed. I am delighted to be so flexible, so relaxed . . . I am happy to be the wife of an interesting and witty man . . . A wonderful sensation of relaxation pervades my body . . . A profound happiness, a great sense of well-being envelops me from head to foot.

"Each day, I experience this pleasant relaxation . . . Day by day, it grows."

I advised her not to stop the hypnosis, by means of the usual appropriate suggestions, but to remain in this state until she awoke naturally. After a few weeks, Mrs. Benner assured me that she no longer suffered from headaches.

A few years went by. Mrs. Benner had once more become a very attractive person. Her migraines seemed definitely consigned to a forgotten past.

What pleased me the most was that her husband, at first opposed to hypnotism, never forgot to mention, at every opportunity, the benefits of self-hypnosis.

HOW TO FREE YOURSELF FROM FEAR AND DEPRESSION BY MEANS OF SELF-HYPNOSIS

Self-hypnosis is meant to eliminate depression and anxiety. I will give you an example.

AN EXAMPLE

Mr. Schlosser was very lucky! He had just been appointed director of the branch of the factory where he was employed. So the Schlosser family moved to the South of Germany! What good fortune! At last, his old dream was going to come true. Since childhood, he wanted to live in a spacious villa, far from the noises of town. His **wife** and children shared his enthusiasm.

A new life began in an isolated house situated some twenty miles from town. Twenty-five miles separated Mr. Schlosser from his place of work! But he was content, happy. The children very quickly grew accustomed to country life.

But it was not so for their mother. Alone all day, left to herself, far from her friends and her usual surroundings, she began to brood. Once every day, she went to the village to do her shopping. But it was by no means enough of a distraction!

Her husband bought her her own car, then a horse. It was all of no use! She withdrew still more into her loneliness. She sat at the window for hours in tears and neglected the house.

I had treated her spouse against tobacco by means of acupuncture. He urged me to attend to his wife. She came to consult me. But because of the distance, I could not undertake a sustained hypnotherapy. I therefore recorded the following suggestion on cassette.

POSITIVE SUGGESTION

"I am quite calm ... Calm, free ... A wonderful feeling of peace and harmony

spreads through my body . . . I feel very happy. I feel quite well in my situation . . . Day by day everything goes better and better . . . Every night, when going to bed, this wonderful feeling of peace and harmony envelops me . . . I fall asleep right away . . . On awakening, I feel fresh, rested . . . From this moment on, I sleep deeply . . . In the mornings, this feeling of peace and harmony surrounds me . . . I am cheerful and happy . . .

"Day by day, I feel better and better . . . I am happier and happier . . . More and more cheerful . . . I feel quite comfortable with my situation . . .

"My assurance and self-confidence grow daily . . . I am happier and happier . . . More and more cheerful . . . I feel quite well."

Mrs. Schlosser was skeptical of her powers. As a result, I obliged her to repeat the suggestions after me.

Note that her depressed feelings were not expressed in them. I explained to her the necessity for this omission.

It is important for positive insinuations, given under self-hypnosis, to take root in the subconscious.

One does not say: "I am not depressed about so and so". This phrase would dictate such feelings to the subconscious, which would definitely absorb them. One instead suggests:

"My head is clear, free of all depression. I feel cheerful and happy".

HOW DO YOU AVOID BECOMING IMPATIENT

Filled with hope, she returned home. Four days later she telephoned me, informing me of her disappointment. The suggestions were ineffective!

I directed her to listen to the cassette for at least thirty days, to give her subconscious the time to react. I advised her not to keep checking on the effect.

I never heard from her again. I had news of her by telephone. Mr. Schlosser, at the other end of the line, reported to me as follows:

"My wife is in town at her dancing lesson. The time of depression has come to an end".

HOW TO BECOME FREE OF ALCOHOLISM BY SELF-HYPNOSIS

A GENUINE ILLNESS

For centuries, alcoholism has been considered a moral weakness. Nowadays, we know that it is an illness. This defect can be corrected by will power, but never eliminated. Has the alcoholic given up his drink? One drink is enough to see him once more the victim!

Only one method is indicated: self-hypnosis, which achieves a complete cure. The sick person must recognize his defect and want to give it up. Under these conditions, the hypnotherapy will be effective.

Mr. Bernhauser came to me for a consultation. Twenty-five years old, his life already seemed to be wasted. A house-painter out of work, his attempts to find work were fruitless. Employers refused to hire someone who, after two weeks, came to work drunk! His driver's license had been taken away for impaired driving. The alcohol level in his bloodstream was 2.5 grams per thousand! His wife and two children left him.

His mother advised him to come to me for a consultation. He hesitated. Two treatments had had no effect. He relapsed after two weeks.

I began to thwart his skepticism by telling him about the actual effectiveness of self-hypnosis. I urged him to abandon his doubts and believe in himself. He was a patient who was hard to convince. He dreamed up every imaginable reason for stopping the treatment. Finally, he agreed to repeat my suggestions, recorded on cassette.

THE SUGGESTION

"I am quite calm ... My breathing is slow, regular ... After each breath, I sink deeper and deeper into a pleasant feeling of tiredness and heaviness ... Deeper and deeper ...

"Nothing distracts me ... A beneficial feeling of tiredness spreads through my body ... My arms and legs are as heavy as lead ... They are becoming heavier and heavier ... As heavy as lead ... Weights seem to be hanging from the ends of them ... Now, I can no longer lift them ... I cannot move them any more ... My arms and legs are quite motionless ... I can no longer raise them ... I no longer want to do so ... With each breath, I surrender more and more to this wonderful feeling of tiredness and heaviness ... I am more and more fatigued ... More and more fa-

tigued . . . With each breath, my fatigue increases still more . . . More and more . . . "

At this point, a minute of silence is observed.

"I feel a great tiredness . . . My body is as heavy as lead . . . I am breathing slowly, regularly . . . I am feeling quite well . . . I feel as if all my problems are going away . . . I will resolve them . . . Nothing will make me change my mind . . . I no longer have any weakness for alcohol . . . Drinking does not interest me any more . . . I find it repugnant . . . More and more . . . The mere thought of alcohol produces this aversion . . . The simple fact of seeing alcohol strengthens my aversion!"

STRENGTHENED SUGGESTIONS

"Now, I will drink no more alcohol . . . Nothing can dissuade me from it . . . I am happy to be instrumental in improving my health . . . Day by day, I feel better and better . . . I will never take another drink . . . My aversion to it in-

creases day by day ... More and more ... The mere thought of alcohol produces disgust ... If I drink a single glass, I will be very ill. All these words are rooted in my subconscious ... I will carry out these commands ... My stomach no longer retains any glass of alcohol ... I would be very ill ... I will try never to give in to temptation ... I will never ... take another drink ... At the very sight of alcohol, my aversion grows and grows ... I am happy to be set free from alcoholism ... Nothing can make me change my conduct ... I can no longer drink alcohol ... I will never drink again!

"Day by day, I feel better and better ... I am happy and proud to have overcome this weakness ... I am free at last ... "

A week later, his mother called me on the telephone. Clearly frantic, she declared, "My son is completely drunk! What can I do?"

I urged her not to abandon him, to encourage him to listen to the cassette at least once a day for three months.

A year went by. Then one day, my patient came to see me, displaying his new driver's license. For a whole year, he had not touched a single drink of alcohol!

HOW TO DETOXIFY DRUG ADDICTS

According to statistics, the percentage of drug addicts is 27% in both urban and rural areas. 17% of them are under twenty-five years of age, and one-third are female.

HOW DOES ONE START TAKING DRUGS?

Narcotics are not restricted to the young. This phenomenon is found in adults of thirty to forty years of age, especially among those who have "made it". The achievement of one's ambitions seems to incite an individual to experience other sensations.

Mr. Hansen (I have changed his name), a professor at the School of Arts and Decoration, began taking drugs after a lesson called, "Art and Drugs". He let himself be drawn into sampling hashish, "To be in the know", and marijuana and L.S.D. followed as a matter of course.

In a few months, he had lost all touch with reality. Dispirited, in despair, out of work, he came to me for a consultation. I suggested various therapeutic procedures.

He replied, "I have lost my self-respect. In order to overcome this feeling, I must conquer my weakness myself. Help me in my affliction".

There was only one way out — self-hypnosis. Together, we developed these suggestions.

THE SUGGESTION

"Now I am closing my eyes, I am relaxing ... Nothing is important anymore ... I surrender completely to this beneficial sensation of relaxation. I feel as if I am becoming more and more detached from real life ... I am freed from my negative, disturbing thoughts ... Nothing is important ... I surrender to the feeling of deliverance ... Everything around me is becoming clear, clean and more and more beautiful ... Colors and music mingle pleasantly ... I surrender to the influence of the sound and color ... Nothing distracts me ... I am indifferent to external noises ... I concentrate on myself ... I attain an ecstasy greater than that from drugs ... I can put myself at will into this state ...

"I will be set free from my cares, my problems and from any bad influence ... No drug could make me experience such

an event . . . I no longer need this drug which is destroying my health . . . Day by day it is improving . . . I have faith in my destiny which I control according to my wishes . . . From now on, nothing can tempt me to take drugs again . . . I don't see the use of it any more . . . Drugs disgust me . . . No power in the world can make me take drugs again . . . If I feel the need to see life through rose-colored glasses, I will use self-hypnosis and meditation . . . My system will be regenerated in this way . . . Day by day, a beneficial influence gives me new strength and the courage to make me look on my fate with optimism . . . I control my destiny according to the mental images that I create of my desires . . . I do not yield to any external influence . . . I am giving a new direction to my life . . . Day by day, I follow the path of my marvelous destiny . . . I am very happy . . . free."

Three minutes of silence.

"I practice a few moments of meditation every day . . . I concentrate on my future

*obligations ... I am brimming with
strength and energy ... Day by day, the
solution to my problems becomes
clearer ... I improve my performance
more and more ... Now, I will count to
three ... On three, I will open my eyes. I
will awaken, brimming with strength
and energy ...*

*"One ... Two ... Three ... I open my
eyes! I am awake, full of strength and
energy ... My arms and legs are once
more flexible and can move ... I feel very
well ... Very well."*

HOW DO YOU GAIN A NEW LEASE ON LIFE?

My patient promised to record this suggestion on cassette and to listen to it several times a day. For weeks, I heard no more of him. I wrote to him. The letter came back to me marked: no longer at this address.

Several months went by in silence. Then, one day, I found a letter in my mailbox. Mr. Hansen had moved into town. He had changed his life, adopted a new personality definitely freed of all craving for drugs.

HOW TO GIVE BIRTH PAINLESSLY WITH THE HELP OF SELF-HYPNOSIS

FEAR LEADS TO CONTRACTIONS, WHICH ARE THE CAUSE OF PAIN

Many women are prone to an unpleasant failing, that of talking about their "difficult delivery". The details, painful and often exaggerated, take root in the subconscious of young women, totally tensed up at the thought of giving birth.

However, it is possible to give birth without pain. It consists of avoiding contractions, which are the cause of pain.

In other words, the fear of suffering creates suffering. If a woman accepts, while relaxed, the idea of childbirth, it will take place quickly and without pain.

Several methods reduce or eliminate suffering. The most effective, nevertheless, is still self-hypnosis. The diminution of pain during childbirth is one of its main effects.

Next, the field of consciousness is reduced so that it has no more idea of the remaining suffering. This too will disappear.

HOW ARE THE CONTRACTIONS REMOVED IN ADVANCE?

Preparation for childbirth by means of hypnosis and self-hypnosis will preferably begin in the sixth month before delivery. It is the way to avoid contractions due to the expectation of contraction, which blocks the necessary relaxation.

Do breathing exercises and record these suggestions on cassette.

THE SUGGESTION

"I am lying down, calm, relaxed ... All my muscles are loose ... All my nerves are relaxed ... I am feeling very well ... Nothing can irritate me ... Now, I am concentrating on my breathing ... I feel absorbed in it ... My breathing is slow, regular ... With each exhalation, I am sinking deeper and deeper into this wonderful feeling of peace and security ... This peacefulness envelops me ... I am feeling very well and very safe ... With each exhalation, I am sinking deeper and deeper into this feeling of peace and security ... "

Here, a minute of silence is observed.

"I am feeling this wonderful peace ... An opening to the subconscious ... This opening is growing wider ... Every suggestion takes root there."

USING THE HAND TO INDUCE HYPNOSIS

"As soon as I look at the palm of my right hand, while lying down, I sink immediately into a pleasant state of peace and security ... It will be enough to lie down and look once at my hand ... All my muscles relax right away ... My nerves are calm ... I will sink into this pleasant state of drowsiness, fatigue and heaviness ... In this state, I feel no more pain ... I feel very well ... I am feeling the contractions, but they cause a pleasant sensation ... With each contraction, I sink into this pleasant state of peace ...

"Nothing is important ... Everything seems very far away ... In this state, I feel an indescribable well-being coming

*over me ... I feel that I am in good
hands."*

A minute of silence is observed.

*"I feel very well and I am waiting impa-
tiently for this birth ... This is all engraved in my subconscious ... As soon
as I look at my right hand, I will sink
into this state of relaxing drowsiness ...
There is no pain ... All I must do is look
at my palm and all pain will disappear ... I feel quite well."*

A minute of silence is observed.

*"This wonderful state of peace grows
deeper and deeper ... Each of my words
is engraved in my subconscious ... It
will carry them out ... Soon, I will count
to three ... On three, I will open my
eyes ... I will be brimming with energy ... Fresh and alert ... One ...
Two ... Three ... My arms and legs are
light once more ... I feel fresh and
alert ... "*

If you listen to this cassette daily, it will be enough for you to look at the inner side of your right hand during delivery. Immediately, you will sink into this second state, strengthened by every pain.

HOW YOU CAN GET RID OF FEAR OF THE DENTIST

The application of hypnosis, or of suggestion in the waking state, allows dentists' patients to eliminate their fear. Self-hypnosis provides them with the means of submitting themselves, relaxed, to treatment.

THE SUGGESTION

Do you have a raging toothache? Are you afraid of the dentist? Prepare for painless treatment with the help of self-hypnosis, in these terms:

"I am quite calm ... Quite calm. My breathing is calm, my breathing is regular ... I am feeling quite well ... Nothing can distract me ... My arms and legs are flexible, relaxed ... I am breathing slowly, regularly ... With each breath, I sink into this pleasant sensation of the peace of relaxation ... This feeling spreads through my body ... With each breath, I surrender still more to this sensation of peace and relaxation ... This feeling covers me like a cloak ... I feel safe, free, relaxed ... I

am feeling quite well . . . I surrender completely to this sensation of peace and security . . . Nothing distracts me . . . I am feeling quite well.

"I am placing around my teeth an invisible steel shield that no pain can get through . . . It is far stronger than novocaine . . . far stronger than laughing gas . . . It numbs my teeth and gums completely . . . No pain can penetrate it . . . It will stay in place no matter how long I am in the dentist's chair . . . I will feel no pain there . . . I am free of pain there . . . I am free of pain until I myself tell myself to take away the invisible shield.

"This wonderful state of peace gives me an opening to my subconscious . . . This opening grows wider . . . All my words take root in my subconscious . . . I will obey these commands".

HOW DO YOU BLOCK ALL THE PATHS OF PAIN?

"As soon as I push my fingernail against the inside of my little finger, I block all the paths of pain* . . . A wonderful feeling of peacefulness and security surrounds me . . . While I push my fingernail against the inside of my little finger, I will be free of all pain . . . I will feel completely well . . . Nothing will distract me . . . There will be steel blocks around my pain centers . . . No pain can get through them . . . They are invulnerable to pain.

"Because of all this, I will feel a pleasant peacefulness and a wonderful sensation of security . . . Besides, as soon as I push my fingernail against the interior face of my little finger, I will be freed of all pain . . . I will feel quite well. This wonderful sensation of peacefulness and security will immediately pervade my body . . . All this is engraved on my subconscious . . . I will carry out all these commands . . . I feel freed from all

fear . . . relaxed . . . I am feeling quite well."

*The point at which pain is blocked is situated on the inner face of the little finger, at the level of the base of the nail. Exert pressure on this spot, on the outer face of the little finger. Bring the fingernail one half inch towards the inside. If you have found the sensitive point, stay on it. It is the point from which you will block pain (See Manuel Pratique de Ji-Jo, ed. Godefroy).

If you listen to this cassette regularly, you will have the means to block pain at will. You will undergo any treatment calmly and in a relaxed fashion.

NOTE: This secret of hypnotic pain-killing is so effective that it should be used ONLY where the cause of the pain is known in advance. Other pain can be a warning signal from your body, and should not be blocked until the cause is fully known.

HYPNOTIZE DISEASE RIGHT OUT OF YOUR BODY

There is a general self-hypnotic command to follow whenever you suffer from any disease. Hypnosis has been used therapeutically to treat the following diseases (among others): allergies, asthma, skin problems, hayfever, migraines, impotence and frigidity, gastro-intestinal problems, heart spasms, indigestion, intestinal spasms, constipation, and many more.

I do not suggest, of course, that you use this self-hypnosis — despite its great power — by itself. Use it, instead, in conjunction with your own doctor or other health practitioner. See how it speeds the power of his or her treatment.

And, of course, if doctors have proven unable to help you, then do not neglect this potent self-remedy.

Record the following suggestions on tape, and play them to yourself once a day, or more, when needed:

"I am resting, calm, relaxed, my eyes closed. My arms and legs are flexible . . . I feel free, relaxed . . . Nothing distracts me . . . I let myself be drawn along . . . I am breathing slowly, regularly . . . I am quite relaxed . . . A wonderful peacefulness envelops my body.

"In this state of peace, I have an opening to my subconscious . . . This opening grows wider . . . More and more . . . My words are settling into my subconscious . . . Are taking root there . . . I will carry out these commands.

"My body is now suffering from (say here the name of the disease) . . . But this disease exists as much in my mind as in my body . . . And my mind can heal it as quickly as any wonder drug ever invented.

"My mind can heal . . . The great power of my unconscious mind can heal . . . For my unconscious mind reaches down to every cell in my body . . . It speaks to every cell in my body . . . It can see every cell in my body . . . It can tell which of those cells have been invaded . . . Which of those cells are ailing . . . Which of those cells need to be healed.

"I am now commanding my mind to seek out those cells that are ailing . . . To find those cells that have been invaded by this disease . . . The germs in these

cells look to my mind like little fires in my cells, trying to burn up the cells and injure me . . . I see those little fires inside my body, but they are nothing but fires . . . And like all fires, they can be put out by the water of my mind.

"Now I tell my mind to create clouds in the cells above those fires . . . These are dark clouds . . . These are rain clouds . . . I can see these clouds clearly . . . They turn the sky dark over the fires, and then they begin to rain . . . The rain pours down out of them . . . Torrents of rain come down out of them . . . Each cell is filled with pure, soft, healing rain.

"Now the rain pours down on the fires in those cells . . . Great floods of rain come down on the fires in those cells . . . The fires turn to wet smoke in the rain . . . The flames of the fires are put out, one by one, by the rain . . . They are washed away, one by one, by the healing rain . . . Now I can see no more flames . . . No more fires . . . No more smoke . . . There is nothing left of the flames or the

fires ... The gentle, healing rain has washed them all away.

"The disease is gone ... All that is left is the pure, healed cell ... Now that the disease has been put out, I can see the cells healing themselves ... I can see them growing stronger and healthier ... Washed clean and young again ... Free from the disease ... Free from pain ... Free from sickness ... Free from weakness ... Free from any chance for the fires to ever start again".

HOW TO FREE YOURSELF FROM HEADACHES WITH THE HELP OF SELF-HYPNOSIS

Record the following suggestions on tape, and play them to yourself whenever you have a tension or circulation or migraine headache, or feel one coming on:

"I am resting, calm, relaxed, my eyes closed. My arms and legs are flexible ... I feel free, relaxed ... Nothing distracts me ... I let myself be drawn along ... I am breathing slowly, regularly ... I am

*quite relaxed ... A wonderful peaceful-
ness envelops my body.*

*"In this state of peace, I have an opening
to my subconscious ... This opening
grows wider ... More and more ... My
words are settling into my subconscious ... Are taking root there ... I will
carry out these commands.*

*"The pain in my head is not real ... I
feel it now, but it will soon go away ... I
will not concentrate on it ... I will not
let it interfere with what I must do ...
Instead, while I am sitting here, I will
concentrate on my hands ... My entire
mind will concentrate on my two
hands ... I will feel them, resting on my
lap ... I will feel how relaxed they
are ... I will feel how comfortable they
are ... I will feel how cool they are.*

*"Now I will feel my two hands as though
I had just put them in a bowl of warm,
pleasant water ... The water is warming
my hands ... Heat is flowing into my
hands ... They are becoming warmer ...
And warmer ... And warmer ... They*

are drawing all the blood out of my head . . . The blood is leaving my head . . . The pain is leaving my head . . . It is flowing down to my hands . . . And the warmth in my heads is burning up that pain . . . Is dissolving that pain . . . Is radiating out that pain from my fingers.

"The pain has now left my head . . . It has gone down to my hands, and it has been drained out by the warmth of my hands through my fingers . . . It is flowing out of my body . . . Every second, it becomes less and less . . . Now there is no longer any pain whatsoever in my head . . . My head is cool and free of pain . . . My head is cool . . . My hands are warm . . . Pain has left my head and my face and my body . . . I am free of pain . . . All I feel is free and good and happy . . . I am myself again. . .I can open my eyes and love the world again".

HOW YOU CAN CONQUER CONSTIPATION

Many people suffer from constipation at the present time. 8% have a bowel movement two to three times daily. 40% do so at least once a day. More than 60% resort to laxatives. However, any medication weakens the intestine and disrupts tissue exchange, especially the metabolism of potassium, essential to each cell.

Seek, therefore, to train your intestine to daily regularity. Feed yourself in a healthy way and you will not have the problems of constipation. If your occupation calls for you to eat in restaurants, you can put your problems right by means of self-hypnosis. Record the following suggestions on cassette. Listen to them at least once a day for several weeks.

HOW TO COMPEL YOUR COLON TO CLEAN ITSELF OUT AT WILL

"I am quite calm and relaxed ... My eyes are closed ... My arms and legs are flexible ... I am breathing slowly, and regularly ... I am more and more tired ... More and more ... I feel an indescribable well-being ... With each breath, I sink more and more ... More and more ... Everything I hear takes root in

*my subconscious . . . I will carry out
these commands.*

*"I have suffered too long from constipa-
tion . . . Too long have I been a slave to
laxatives . . . Now I am about to break
out of that slavery forever . . . Now I am
about to take natural control of my bowels and my bowel habits . . . Now I am
about to achieve a natural regularity,
every day, when I want it.*

*"My mind now is penetrating deeper and
deeper into my body . . . My mind is
reaching into the middle of my body . . .
My mind is beginning to establish con
trol over all my intestines . . . I can now
feel these intestines, from the bottom of
my stomach to the point where they
leave my body . . . I can feel their
warmth . . . I can feel their strength . . . I
can feel the cleansing power they have
for all my body.*

*"They are my body's cleanser . . . They
are my body's purifier . . . They keep me
well and strong . . . They are well and
strong . . . They want to cleanse my body*

every day . . . They want to take out of
my body every scrap of waste and toxins
that are naturally within them . . . I can
feel their ability to do this . . . I can feel
their strength to do this . . . They are
waiting for my command.

"Every day at this time, they will auto-
matically cleanse themselves com-
pletely . . . Every day at this time, they
will begin to contract and make them-
selves ready for this cleansing expul-
sion . . . Every day at this time, their
urge to cleanse themselves will become
more and more imperative, till there is
nothing I can do to stop them . . . They
will force me into the bathroom for this
daily cleansing . . . Everything will be
perfectly natural, and easy, and com-
fortable . . . There will be no straining . . .
There will be no pain . . . There will be
no irritation of my hemmorhoids.

"Everything will come out without my
having to force it . . . It will be so natu-
ral . . . So easy . . . So irresistible . . . So
painless . . . So strainless . . . And I will
feel so relieved afterwards . . . So much

thinner and lighter . . . So much more in control . . . I will know that every day my bowels will take over the job of cleansing themselves automatically . . . Of making my body clean, and healthy and strong . . . Automatically."

SUBJECTIVE RELAXATION

"From this moment, I will feel obliged to go to the bathroom every morning after breakfast . . . I will not be able to do otherwise . . . I will be obliged to go to the bathroom . . . At night, before going to bed, I will go to the bathroom . . . Once there, all my tension will drain away . . . My stools are normal . . . My colon is compelled to clean itself out . . . To empty itself . . . To rid itself of all the toxins that have poisoned it for all these years . . . Their discharge is easy.

"All tension has disappeared . . . My digestion is excellent . . . Nothing can disrupt it . . . In every situation my digestive functions are excellent . . . I am

happy to have digestive problems no longer . . . I am feeling very well."

A cassette such as this is easily carried on trips. In a short time your constipation will be no more than a bad memory.

HOW TO BECOME YOUNG AND BEAUTIFUL BY MEANS OF SELF-HYPNOSIS

Rare is the person able to pass before a mirror without looking into it. Some admire themselves on the sly, as if this act were shameful. However, it is justifiable to look after our external appearance. It takes the place of our "visiting card". First impressions are often decisive.

HOW YOU CAN STAY YOUNG AT ANY AGE

An attractive appearance and good health are not just attributes of the young. I know many seventy-year-olds who display both of these envious qualities!

"The real age is the one you look like." Our psychic behavior, the sum of our thoughts, constitutes its essential element. The saying, "Thoughts are free," is false. We can express a thought, but we are subject to its effects. Each thought forges a portion of our destiny, our appearance and our youth.

What is the sure, harmless way to become young and beautiful? Self-hypnosis.

It achieves the ancient dream of eternal youth. Self-hypnosis is none other than this fountain of youth from which we draw the secret of the power to improve our external appearance by changing our psychic behavior. The body straightens. The bearing becomes limber, assured. The gaze will be clear and candid. Under self-hypnosis, you can quicken the growth of your hair, make your skin younger and develop your breasts.

HOW TO COMMAND YOUR FACE TO FIRM UP

Record the following suggestions on tape, and play them to yourself once a day:

> "I am resting, calm, relaxed, my eyes closed. My arms and legs are flexible . . . I feel free, relaxed . . . Nothing distracts me . . . I let myself be drawn along . . . I am breathing slowly, regularly . . . I am quite relaxed . . . A wonderful peaceful-ness envelops my body.

> "In this state of peace, I have an opening to my subconscious . . . This opening grows wider . . . More and more . . . My words are settling into my subcon-scious . . . Are taking root there . . . I will carry out these commands.

"At this moment, I will concentrate on my face ... I will first feel every muscle in my face ... I will let my head lean back, as though I were resting in a purifying, harmless sun ... My face becomes warm ... Every muscle in it becomes warm ... As the warmth spreads throughout my face, I feel the outline of every muscle ... I can feel the complete control I am gaining over each of those muscles.

"Now I will drain the tiredness out of those muscles ... I am gently commanding the muscles in my face to reward themselves ... To lose their tension ... To glow with new energy and youth ... I can feel the fatigue drain out of them ... I can feel the youth pour into them ... I can feel my face growing younger and younger and younger.

"Now every muscle in my face is wonderfully relaxed ... In this relaxed state, it has no more resistance to my commands for it ... When I now tell it to grow firmer, it will obey at once ... I tell the muscles of my face to grow firmer ... All

*the muscles of my face to grow firmer all
at once ... I feel my face begin to lift itself ... I feel the muscles of my face begin move gently up and back toward my
hair ... I feel the gentle tightening and
tingling in my chin area ... I feel the
skin around my cheek bones rise and
rise ... I feel the skin around my eyes
tighten and begin to erase the crow's feet
surrounding them.*

*"My face is beginning to grow young
again ... The skin of my face is beginning to grow firm again ... The mis-
takes that age made in my face are
beginning to be forgiven by my mind ...
I am gaining control over my face ... I
am happy ... I am delighted".*

HOW TO COMMAND YOUR HAIR
TO GROW FULLER

Record the following suggestions on tape, and play
them to yourself once a day:

*"I am resting, calm, relaxed, my eyes
closed. My arms and legs are flexible ...
I feel free, relaxed ... Nothing distracts*

me . . . I let myself be drawn along . . . I am breathing slowly, regularly . . . I am quite relaxed . . . A wonderful peacefulness envelops my body.

"*In this state of peace, I have an opening to my subconscious . . . This opening grows wider . . . More and more . . . My words are settling into my subconscious . . . Are taking root there . . . I will carry out these commands.*

"*I run my hand through my hair . . . I feel the softness of my hair . . . Now I lay my hand down, and let my mind take command of my hair . . . I feel the roots of that hair growing like wonderful plants out of my scalp . . . I feel the blood coursing through those roots into that hair . . . I open those roots wider and wider . . . More blood flows through them into my hair . . . I can feel more blood running through them into my hair . . . I can feel that blood feeding my hair . . . Pouring new strength, new power, new growth into that hair.*

"Minute by minute, my hair is becoming thicker and thicker . . . Fuller and fuller . . . It now glows with a beautiful shimmer . . . More and more of it springs up from my scalp . . . Where there was little or no hair before, old roots regain thier youthful power . . . I am delighted . . . My hair is once more becoming my crowning glory".

HOW CAN YOU DEVELOP YOUR BREASTS?

Recently, I read the following in a magazine: Doctors James E. Williams and M. S. Gregg-Harrison of Texas succeeded in expanding the chests of nineteen women. They were increased by two inches.

These facts called to mind an experiment I had performed before a group of physicians. Skeptical, they refused to admit the following theory: the physical system of the body can be penetrated and influenced by suggestion. Thanks to hypnosis, the atrophied breasts of an adult woman will expand.

I made the attempt with a student, twenty-two years old. Distressed by a chest that was quite flat, she willingly submitted to the experiment. I proceeded in the following manner.

With the patient's permission, I started the experiment on the right breast. I did this to prove the effectiveness of hypnosis. I suggested:

> *"Your right breast will grow larger day by day ... But your left breast will not change".*

And that is exactly what happened. The subject, amazed at her success, begged me to continue the treatment.

In two weeks her left breast was as big as the right one.

HOW YOU CAN DO THE SAME

Record the following suggestions on tape, and play them to yourself once a day:

> *"I am resting, calm, relaxed, my eyes closed. My arms and legs are flexible ... I feel free, relaxed ... Nothing distracts me ... I let myself be drawn along ... I am breathing slowly, regularly ... I am quite relaxed ... A wonderful peacefulness envelops my body.*

> *"In this state of peace, I have an opening to my subconscious ... This opening*

grows wider . . . More and more . . . My words are settling into my subconscious . . . Are taking root there . . . I will carry out these commands.

"My breasts are now about to become the full, feminine size they were meant to be, that I have always wanted them to be . . . They are going to become firmer and larger and more beautiful in a perfectly natural way.

"I will start with the left breast . . . I will feel warmth radiating down from my mind into it . . . It will be as though I were laying on a beautiful beach, on a blanket, surrounding by pure white sand . . . The sun sits above me, filling my body and my breast with soothing warmth . . . I have put on suntan lotion, so there is no threat . . . Only the purifying, growing, gentle rays of the sun.

"My left breast is becoming warmer and warmer . . . As I lay there, I can feel it begin to gently expand in the warmth of the sun . . . I can feel it begin to capture the nourishment of the sun, and gently

*grow firmer and larger . . . I am re-
laxed . . . I am calm . . . I am happy.*

*"Now the sun begins to warm my right
breast as well . . . Both breasts are now
being warmed and nourished by the
sun . . . Both are gently firming and expanding . . . I am becoming more of the
woman I have always dreamed of . . . I
am becoming more beautiful, more attractive, more self-confident . . . My
breasts will continue to expand until I
am fully satisfied with their size and
shape . . . I am so warm . . . I am so
happy . . . I am so grateful to myself".*

HOW TO QUIET A CHILD'S BLADDER
SO HE CAN SLEEP
FOR 8 HOURS WITHOUT THE SLIGHTEST
BED-WETTING PROBLEM

Record the following suggestions on tape, and play
them to your child once a night, just after he or she goes
to sleep:

*"I am resting, calm, relaxed, my eyes
closed. My arms and legs are flexible . . .
I feel free, relaxed . . . Nothing distracts*

me . . . I let myself be drawn along . . . I am breathing slowly, regularly . . . I am quite relaxed . . . A wonderful peacefulness envelops my body.

"In this state of peace, I have an opening to my mind . . . This opening grows wider . . . More and more . . . My words are settling into my mind . . . Are taking root there . . . I will carry out these commands.

"From this moment on, wetting my bed when I am asleep will be a memory from the past . . . No matter how much I have done this before, it will not happen again . . . There is no need for it to happen again, because from now on my bladder will go to sleep with me . . . It will be numb all night . . . It not feel itself getting full . . . It will not have the need to empty itself . . . Not a single drop will leak out . . . It will be as quiet as I am quiet . . . It will sleep as soundly as I sleep . . . All night long, it will sleep as soundly as I sleep . . . And when I wake up in the morning, my bed will be

dry . . . I will be dry . . . I will be so proud
of myself . . . I will be so happy".

And remember, during this most peaceful sleep, you can "suggest away" thumb sucking, loss of appetite, even personality disorders such as laziness, lying, cowardliness, etc.

INFLUENCING A VITAL FUNCTION WITH THE MIND

Each second of our lives, innumerable cells perish. Others take their place. Here is the way to influence this function at will: self-hypnosis.

Do you want your entire body to become young and beautiful? Do you want the cells of your body to self-rejuvenate? Then record the following suggestions on cassette.

THE SUGGESTIONS

"I am quite calm . . . I am closing my
eyes and relaxing . . . Nothing can dis-
tract me . . . Nothing is important . . . All
my muscles are relaxed . . . My nerves
are quite relaxed . . . I feel as though I
am detached from reality . . . I surrender

to this beneficial relaxation ... I am feeling very well ... I am concentrating on my breathing ... With each exhalation I sink deeper and deeper into this wonderful sensation of peace and security ... I surrender to this feeling of freedom ... This wonderful peace and this security cover me like a cloak ... I am feeling well ... Nothing is important anymore ... I open myself totally to the following suggestions:

"I am quite calm ... Free ... A wonderful sensation of peace and harmony surrounds me ... Fills me ... Nothing else has any importance ... I surrender altogether to this feeling of peace and harmony ... I am very happy ... I feel comfortable in my situation ... I look to the future with confidence ... I know beautiful happenings await me ... My heart beats slowly, evenly. My circulation is regular ... Calm, regular ... My digestion is excellent ... Day by day, my health improves and day by day, everything is going better".

ACCEPTING YOUR SITUATION

"I accept my situation and I am quite comfortable with it . . . My head is light . . . The nape of my neck and my shoulders are flexible and relaxed . . . I experience this wonderful relaxation throughout my body . . . I am pleased with this sense of well-being which spreads through my body . . . I enjoy a deep, beneficial, restful sleep . . . Every night, I sleep without awakening . . . Every morning, I awaken fresh, rested . . . I rejoice to be able to live a new day . . . I contemplate the future with confidence . . . Each new day fills me with joy . . . My health improves day by day . . . I get even slimmer . . . I am happy to be so comfortable . . . Day by day, there is improvement in every way . . . My skin becomes taut . . . I am becoming younger and younger . . . Slimmer and slimmer . . . A new, unknown energy pervades me . . . I follow all my problems joyfully . . . I have taken my fate in hand . . . I shape it to my desires . . . I give the desired shape to my life . . . I am very happy."

A minute of silence is observed here.

ATTAINING PERFECT RELAXATION

"I feel this wonderful relaxation . . . It fills my body . . . Day by day, it floods over me still more . . . In this wonderful state of peace and relaxation, each cell of my body is filled with new strength . . . The poisons are draining out of it . . . It is growing younger and stronger every moment . . . I am full of strength and energy . . . I am feeling very well . . . Soon, I am going to count to three . . . Then I will open my eyes once more . . . I will be fresh and alert . . . One . . . Two . . . Three . . . I open my eyes! Now my arms and legs are once more flexible, capable of motion . . . I am brimming with strength and energy and I am feeling fresh and alert . . . I am feeling very well."

You will be surprised by the effect achieved. Listen to these suggestions twice a day for more than a month.

HOW TO BREAK THE CHILDHOOD CHAINS THAT BIND YOU TO THE ERRORS OF THE PAST

Record the following suggestions on tape, and play them to yourself whenever you feel the need:

"I am resting, calm, relaxed, my eyes closed. My arms and legs are flexible . . . I feel free, relaxed . . . Nothing distracts me . . . I let myself be drawn along . . . I am breathing slowly, regularly . . . I am quite relaxed . . . A wonderful peacefulness envelops my body.

"In this state of peace, I have an opening to my subconscious . . . This opening grows wider . . . More and more . . . My words are settling into my subconscious . . . Are taking root there . . . I will carry out these commands.

"Today I acted as though I were a child again . . . I gave in to childhood fears and fantasies . . . I trapped myself in the past, and did not allow myself to grow into the future . . . I will not do that again.

"My eyes are closed . . . My mind is open . . . The past I suffered from as a child is completely available to me . . . I will go into that past now . . . I will go into that past in order to forgive it . . . In order to forgive myself . . . In order to forgive my parents . . . In order to forgive all those who hurt me then . . . And, in forgiving them, free myself from them at last.

"I felt today as though I were a child again . . . I felt those childhood fears . . . I felt as though, if I did what I wanted, I would be punished as a child . . . As I was punished when I was a child . . . But now I realize that those people who punished me then are gone . . . They were powerful then, but they are not powerful now . . . They have died, or they have grown older, or they are far, far away . . . They can no longer control me, because I forgive them . . . And I forgive me . . . And, by forgiving, I make myself free.

"I am an adult now . . . I am no longer a child, but an adult . . . I am free now . . . I am free of these old childhood feel-

*ings . . . I am free of this old childhood
fear . . . I am free of this old childhood
feeling of not being good enough . . . I am
free to do as I want, now, as an adult.*

*"The next time I feel panic like this . . .
The next time I feel fear like this . . . I
will automatically pause . . . I will
automatically feel the panic drain out of
my body . . . I will automatically feel the
fear drain out of my body . . . I will look
at what's happening with adult eyes . . . I
will react to what's happening as an
adult, and not as a child . . . I will feel
the panic, and then I will put it aside . . .
I will feel the fear, and then I will put it
aside. . . . I will be able at last to try new
things . . . To open myself to the
future . . . To become the person I've
always dreamed of . . . To grow and dare
and love and enjoy".*

HOW TO SUCCEED IN YOUR LOVE LIFE BY MEANS OF SELF-HYPNOSIS

IS HAPPINESS POSSIBLE WITHOUT A SUCCESSFUL LOVE LIFE?

Even while abstaining from most of life's ordinary rewards, a person can be perfectly happy. But without a successful love life, all of life seems nonsensical.

What bars us from the love we all deserve? Usually one bad experience — a rejection, or an unhappy love affair — is responsible for a vicious circle of negative conditioning.

Once the infernal circle is closed, one gives in to it by calling it "fate".

In such a case, the circle must be broken. Under self-hypnosis, you will relive "positive" romantic events until the habit of success in your love life is acquired.

It makes no difference whether these "events" are fictional or real. Either way, their very image, intensified by the hypnotic process, will be enough to arouse the feeling of being able to succeed in gaining the one you are attracted to in the future.

THE TECHNIQUE OF THE MENTAL IMAGE

Relive your most beautiful erotic scene under self-hypnosis. Do you not remember any? Then imagine one according to your wildest dreams. Repeat it. Your reactions will take root in your subconscious, will be identified with your personality.

How do you go about it?

Start by putting yourself under self-hypnosis with the aid of the usual suggestions. Describe the erotic scenes in detail, aloud. Say, for instance, "My psychic eye sees that I ... etc."

Follow this with an exact description of events. Once this is finished, observe two to three minutes of silence. You will end the self-hypnosis in these terms.

THE SUGGESTIONS

"This event is engraved in my subconscious ... In future, I will react in the same way ... Now, I will count to three ... On three, I will open my eyes, I will be completely awake and in good health ... My body is brimming with strength and energy. One ... Two ... Three ... I open my eyes! ... I am completely awake and I feel fresh and alert!"

If you wish, you may add a global suggestion to your description. Here are a few examples to be adapted to your situation:

"When I take my partner in my arms, an irresistible desire overcomes me ... I am ready to go into action ... Physical love is quite natural ... I do it while relaxed, without any complexes ... I am happy to be with my partner ... The mere idea is enough to stimulate this desire which overruns my body ... I am ready for love".

Similar suggestions have helped many to a complete fulfillment in the sphere of love.

HOW TO GET RID OF STRESS WITH SELF-HYPNOSIS

TRAINING YOUR SYSTEM

This indispensable training drills your body to withstand overwork until an advanced age. It is not the extent of stress that we cannot endure, but the degree of overwork it creates.

This training relieves this. This is the secret of people practicing joyously — and without feeling the least fatigue — an occupation that would give others a heart attack in a few days.

This training consists of reliving such situations under self-hypnosis. In it, you will imagine that you master them, calm, sure of yourself, enveloped in a pleasant sensation of peace.

This self-education under hypnosis will give you an endurance that will meet the test of any situation. You will acquire the certainty of being the victor while keeping your composure, a factor in having a long life.

ANTI-STRESS SUGGESTIONS

"I am lying comfortably and I am closing my eyes . . . All my muscles are loosened and my nerves are relaxed . . . I am feeling very well . . . Nothing can distract me, nothing is important . . . I surrender to this sensation of peace and security . . . My breathing is slow, even . . . I am completely relaxed and I am feeling very well . . . With each breath, I sink deeper and deeper into this pleasant feeling of tiredness and heaviness . . . I am more and more tired . . . More and more."

A minute of silence is observed here.

"My peace is profound . . . In this wonderful state of peace, I have an opening to my subconscious . . . This opening is getting bigger . . . All these words are definitely engraved on my subconscious . . . I will obey these commands . . .

"I am quite calm . . . Relaxed . . . I will concentrate on everything I do and I will remain calm and relaxed internally . . . I will perform my task in a calm and re-

laxed manner ... Nothing can make me lose my composure ... I know that I will be the victor in every situation ... This certainty fills me with strength and energy ... I am sure of myself ... It is a wonderful feeling to be able to say, I shall overcome! I complete all my projects calm and relaxed ... Day by day, my peace and self-assurance increase ... I am calmer and calmer ... I feel quite at ease ... My heart beats calmly, evenly ... My circulation is regular ... Each effort makes me stronger and stronger ... My health improves daily ... I sleep deeply ... As soon as I am in bed, all my problems go away ... I fall asleep right away ... My sleep is healthy, natural, acts as a tonic ... In the morning, I awaken rested, happy for the day just beginning ... I feel quite at ease ... Day by day, everything gets better and better ... I feel better ... "

Three minutes of silence are observed here.

HOW IS A SENSE OF WELL-BEING INDUCED?

"I surrender joyfully to this sense of well-being which pervades me from head to foot . . . I experience again this wonderful relaxation which pervades my body . . . In this peace, each cell of my body is filled with strength and energy . . . I am feeling very well . . . Soon, I will count to three. On three, I will open my eyes . . . I will be brimming with strength and energy . . . I will feel fresh and alert . . . One . . . Two . . . Three . . . My arms and legs are once more flexible, light, capable of motion . . . I feel fresh and alert."

Once this is recorded on tape, listen to it regularly; you will eventually be able to make any effort without being the victim of overwork.

HOW TO IMPROVE PERFORMANCE IN SPORTS WITH THE HELP OF SELF-HYPNOSIS

More and more athletes resort to self-hypnosis to improve their athletic performance. A book has been devoted to the subject: *How You Can Play Better Golf, Using Self-Hypnosis*, by Jack Heise, Willshire Book Company, publishers.

To what extent does self-hypnosis influence people's performance? I will give you several conclusive examples.

SAMPLE EXPERIMENTS

The muscular energy of several people was measured. It amounted to one hundred grams. Then the suggestion of tiredness and weakness was made to them. The energy level diminished by 70 grams. Next, it was suggested that they possessed a herculean strength. The muscular energy immediately increased by 50 grams.

I myself have carried out such experiments.

A weight-lifter came to me for consultation. I told him of the powers of self-hypnosis. He asked me, "Can one's athletic performance be improved under hypnosis?"

At that time, I did not know the answer. But I was quite willing to try the experiment. I went to see him training to lift heavier and heavier weights. Suddenly, he gave up. The next weight seemed to be beyond his normal ability. I gave him the suggestion:

"Your energy is at its maximum . . . an unknown strength envelops you".

Several minutes went by. He lifted the weight he had given up on, then two more.

In ten minutes, he had improved his performance by 11.2%.

Dr. William S. Kroger, an enthusiastic supporter of the application of hypnosis to the improvement of athletic performance, relates identical experiments carried out at the University of Illinois.

To one athlete, who specialized in running, he administered a placebo (a palliative and hypnotic medication. It contains no active elements. The effect is produced subjectively by suggestion.) and ordered him:

"This medicine improves your performance . . . You will outdo your colleague".

And the athelete triumphed over his competitor in every race. Next, Dr. Kroger made his adversary swallow a placebo while suggesting to him:

"In a short time, you will regain your superiority".

And he did!

The two athletes had clearly improved their performance by this procedure. This acquired behavior survived in the future.

NO DANGER OF OVERWORK

Dr. Michiki Ikai, professor of philology at the University of Tokyo, studied these phenomena. He put forward the conclusion: there is no danger of physical excess through improving performance under hypnosis or self-hypnosis. Only inhibitions are eliminated in this way — only the hidden obstacles to surpassing yourself.

Dr. Kroger and Dr. Ikai assert:

"Involuntary reflexes of the athlete's system preserve him from the dangers of overwork".

It must not be forgotten that high-ranking athletic performance is not achieved only by strength. Other essential factors come into play: physical and mental condition, single-mindedness in attaining one's goal and an unshakeable faith in victory.

Do you want to improve your athletic performance? Bring the positive suggestions together in one global suggestion.

Then insert personal suggestions into the paragraphs, wherever you feel they are called for.

THE SUGGESTIONS

"Now, I am closing my eyes . . . I am relaxing. I feel a wonderful peace entering my body . . . Nothing can distract me . . . Nothing is important . . . I surrender completely to this wonderful sensation of peace and relaxation . . . I am breathing slowly, regularly . . . I am quite relaxed . . . I am feeling quite well . . . With each breath, I sink deeper and deeper into this beneficial sensation of fatigue and heaviness . . . I am more and more tired . . . More and more tired."

A minute of silence is observed here.

"My peace is profound . . . Nothing can distract me . . . I feel light . . . I no longer feel my arms and legs . . . I am transparent, airborne . . . Everything is light,

free . . . I surrender completely to the ef-
fect of the following suggestions. Each
word enters my subconscious . . . Defi-
nitely takes root there . . . I will carry out
these commands . . . My heart beats
calmly, evenly . . . even effortlessly . . . My
circulation is regular . . . My cardiac
muscle is strong . . . I feel at ease in ac-
complishing an effort . . . I am able to
provide any effort at all . . . I am
stronger and stronger . . . In every situa-
tion, my head is clear . . . All complexes
have definitely disappeared . . . I am
flexible, free . . . Ready to give of my
best . . . I feel as if this wonderful relax-
ation fills my body . . . Day by day, this
relaxation increases."

INDIVIDUAL SUGGESTIONS

"My sleep is becoming deeper and
deeper . . . Deeper and deeper . . . I re-
joice in all competition for I know that
my performance improves day by
day . . . Day by day, my performance
improves . . . I am feeling very well . . . "

Three minutes of silence are observed here.

"This wonderful relaxation once more fills my body . . . I feel this pleasant relaxation which envelops me more and more . . . A tremendous strength envelops my whole body . . . each of my cells is filled with new strength . . . I am brimming with strength and energy and I am ready to give my best at any time . . . I am feeling very well . . . Soon, I will count to three . . . I will open my eyes . . . I will be completely awake, fresh and alert . . . One . . . Two . . . Three . . . I open my eyes! I am completely awake and I feel fresh and alert . . . My arms and legs are once more light and capable of movement . . . I am full of energy . . . I feel quite well."

With the help of this cassette, you will rid yourself of your complexes. You will be ready to give of your best at any time.

HOW YOU CAN IMPROVE YOUR INTELLIGENCE AND INSPIRATION

AMAZING EXPERIMENTS

Experiments performed at the neuro-psychiatric clinic in Moscow prove that hypnosis has a positive influence on human ability and raises the intellectual level.

Professor W. Raikow put 150 graduates and 50 students under deep hypnosis. They remained in this state for four weeks. All of a sudden, they displayed amazing gifts for pottery decoration and for glass-blowing.

The faculty of observation increases under hypnosis. The candidates' memory of two hundred foreign words and their translations was more accurate then in in the waking state. The posthypnotic effect lasted four to twelve weeks, but then could be renewed.

If you regularly suggest a light hypnosis lasting seven days, at the end of a year you will obtain an improvement in intelligence. This will be from 1.5 to 2.5 times higher than the intellectual level in the normal state!

A surprising creative and energetic force seems to be developed under hypnosis and under self-hypnosis. Professor Magnin tells of his patient, Madeleine, in his book — *Kunst und Hypnose*. Madeleine, temperamental and unbalanced in the normal state, became a talented artist under hypnosis. Her flawless dancing and mime, independent of any prompting, guided by excellent music, won the acclaim of the most severe critics.

Under hypnosis, you can develop a gift for languages. The study of a foreign language certainly requires the memory, but above all, it demands a great faculty of concentration.

HOW TO SKYROCKET THE POWER OF YOUR MIND

Record the following suggestions on tape, and play them to yourself once a day:

"I am resting, calm, relaxed, my eyes closed. My arms and legs are flexible . . . I feel free, relaxed . . . Nothing distracts me . . . I let myself be drawn along . . . I am breathing slowly, regularly . . . I am quite relaxed . . . A wonderful peacefulness envelops my body.

"In this state of peace, I have an opening to my subconscious . . . This opening grows wider . . . More and more . . . My

words are settling into my subconscious . . . Are taking root there . . . I will carry out these commands.

"So far, I have been using only a small fraction of the true power of my mind . . . I have been using only 5 or 10 percent of the true power of my mind . . . Now I will begin to use more and more of it . . . Now I will begin to use it all".

Let a moment of silence pass.

"When I need to learn something . . . when I need to study . . . I will then automatically block all other thoughts from my mind . . . My mind will be filled only with what I need to learn . . . Every thing else will disappear for that moment from my mind . . . I will think only about what it is that I have to learn . . . I will open my mind to it like a great video camera . . . I will automatically take all of it in . . . I will automatically record it on my memory like a video camera records everything it sees and hears.

"I will think only about what it is I have to learn . . . I will think about nothing else . . . My full mind will be devoted to taking it in . . . To recording it on my memory . . . To be able to call it back to my full mind anytime I wish . . . All my memories will now become available to me anytime I wish . . . All of them will be ready to spring into my mind whenever I need them . . . I can use all of them to pass whatever tests life may give me . . . To solve new problems . . . To create new, winning ideas.

"I have the high-powered mind I have always dreamed of . . . I can think now with the best of them . . . I can learn huge new vocabularies . . . I no longer have to be ashamed of my mind or my background or my memory . . . I can be with the people I want to be with . . . I can talk with them . . . I can make them respect and listen to me and follow me . . . I can have the mind I have always wanted . . . to give me the life I have always wanted."

THE TRUE SUGGESTIONS OF JOY

It's easy to concentrate on an interesting subject. Do you intend to learn a foreign language? Then give yourself the following suggestion:

"Day by day, the study of this language pleases me still more . . . I await each new lesson with impatience".

Increase your concentration by the suggestion:

"I am concentrating exclusively on the study of this foreign language . . . Nothing can distract me . . . Each of my words is definitely engraved in my subconscious . . . I will forget nothing that I have learned".

In order to bring to a successful conclusion some work that demands creativity and inspiration, suggest to yourself under self-hypnosis:

"The necessary inspiration will come to me during sleep . . . Tomorrow, I will resolve all my problems as a matter of course".

Have faith in your subjective reserves and give yourself the needed suggestions, free of all possible doubts. Be convinced of obtaining a positive result. Under these conditions, your subconscious will be your most trustworthy ally.

HOW IS SELF-HYPNOSIS INDUCED BY THE HYPNOSIS OF OTHERS?

Many people wish to make use of the power of self-hypnosis. But they do not persevere in practicing it. So, they achieve no results.

In such a case, recourse must be made to the hypnosis of others. The hypnotist will establish a rapport by which he transfers the desired command to himself. With the person hypnotized, he will agree on a word which will induce deep hypnosis. Then, he will suggest to him:

"You will carry out every command that you express in thought under self-hypnosis, as if it came to you from myself".

One single hypnosis is necessary. It allows one to proceed immediately to self-hypnosis.

THE TECHNIQUE OF IMAGINATION

This method, little known but very effective, deserves to be mentioned in this chapter.

I affirm yet again:

The hypnosis of others and self-hypnosis do not require extraordinary powers.

The conviction that excellent results can only be achieved under deep hypnosis is erroneous. Light hypnosis will do.

Why? Because the technique of imagination allows you to deepen that light hypnosis. Your psychic eye sees you sinking more and more deeply into the hypnotic state.

Soon, under the influence of these repeated light hypnoses, you will be in a state of deep hypnosis where all things are possible to you.

Practice! Learn! Achieve more and more control over yourself and others!

Hypnosis and self-hypnosis are the keys to the life you have always dreamed of. Everything you need is in these four volumes. I wish you the incredible results I know you deserve.

SUMMARY

THE LAWS OF HYPNOSIS

If you want to practice hypnosis successfully, you must know its laws. Once understood, their methodical application will govern your success. I have already explained them to you in one chapter. Given their importance, I would like to recapitulate.

FIRST LAW

Every mental image which you allow to take complete control of your mind tends to be realized.

Nothing physical in this world can be created, nor can be destroyed by man. We can only give another shape to things.

Nevertheless, our thoughts do not follow this rule. We can create a thought.

Coming from nowhere, this wonderful creative activity causes reflection. Nothing we want to do in this world is conceivable without such creative thought. This therefore represents the essential part of our creative faculty. And the practical, automatic realization of our desires follows from it.

Every idea can be realized IF ONLY you will make a mental image of it. This mental image can then be powered by the desire that it be realized. And, propelled by that power, it will take concrete form.

Nonetheless, you must observe the following rule:

Nothing in your mind should be in opposition to the mental image you wish to bring about at that moment.

If two mental images, two thoughts, are in opposition, they will neutralize each other.

Here is an example: the mental image of sleep causes sleep. But the mental image of insomnia produces insomnia.

If you allow them to exist in your mind at the same time, they will cancel out be other. You will do nothing — gain nothing.

We have there the effect of the second law.

SECOND LAW

If will and conviction are opposed, conviction will prevail.

Who does not want to go to sleep in his bed at night? But if you are "convinced" that you won't be able to sleep, you won't find sleep in spite of your opposing "will" to fall asleep.

This is a simple application of this second law. Most people don't even know it. Each of them wishes to be healed. But the one who is *convinced* of it is the only one who will be healed.

This is the secret of miraculous cures. But you must be aware that the opposite effect can also happen. We have seen a person who was thought by physicians to be in good health waste away, then die. Why? Because death met his expectations — for he was convinced of the incurability of his illness.

If you know how to work with this reality, you will become master of your fate. Ineffective desires are rare. Despite a fierce will, most of us do not attain our objective.

He who succeeds knows this law: If will and conviction are opposed, it is conviction that will win out. And he who succeeeds makes this law work for his own good.

He concentrates exclusively on the mental image of his goal — the conscious carrier of his conviction — and avoids all opposing effort. This is the wisdom of the third law.

THIRD LAW

Effort alone produces the reverse of the hoped-for effect.

All voluntary effort to reach your goal without the help of a vivid, detailed, believable mental image is fruitless.

You cannot leave your thoughts and wishes at the abstract level. You cannot vaguely want something, and get it.

To work as you want it to work, each of your thoughts and wishes must exert a very precise and detailed mental influence. It is necessary to control them, to discipline, to vivify them, to be able to make them real in the outside world.

If you have properly understood these three laws, you will succeed with every hypnosis.

IN WHAT CASES IS HYPNOSIS NOT ADVISABLE?

There are cases where hypnosis is not applicable. A distinction is made between absolute contra-indications and relative contra-indications.

ABSOLUTE CONTRA-INDICATIONS

You cannot use hypnotherapy in these cases: schizophrenia, epilepsy, endogenic psychoses, senile weakness of mind.

RELATIVE CONTRA-INDICATIONS

Hypnosis is not advisable in these cases: hypotonia, religious objections, lack of receptivity, pronounced tendency to make only token efforts, a very high rate of defective intelligence.

CONCLUSION

ASSURANCE ACQUIRED THROUGH EXPE-RIENCE

Every practitioner of hypnosis will certify that success depends on your feeling of certainty, of "I can".

This faith in your abilities is not acquired by a simple reading of a system. Your assurance and experience will only be developed with practice. Your successes there will forge the indispensable confidence in yourself.

Live your life, above all, through positive thoughts. Many people are available to influence your life. Control them, and they will give you your destiny. Your life will automatically be transformed by them.

To summarize: only *the practice* of the knowledge contained in this system allows you to fashion your new, positive destiny.

Notes

Notes

Notes

Notes

Notes

Notes

Notes

Notes

Notes

Notes

Notes

Notes

Notes

Notes